TAKING CONTROL

*A Collection of Inspiring Stories for People Living
With Multiple Sclerosis*

By Jillian Kingsford Smith

Taking Control: A Collection of Inspiring Stories for People Living With Multiple Sclerosis

Copyright © 2013 Jillian Kingsford Smith
1st published 2013 by Take20 Stories, Brisbane Qld Australia
www.take20stories.com

Liability Disclaimer: The material contained in this book is general in nature and does not represent professional advice. It is not intended to provide specific guidance for particular circumstances and it should not be relied on as a basis for any decisions to take action on any matter that it covers. Readers should obtain professional advice before acting on any information in this book. Neither the Author nor the Publisher can be held responsible for any loss or claim arising out of the use, or misuse, of the suggestions made or the failure to take medical advice.

National Library of Australia Cataloguing-in-publication data:

Author:	Kingsford-Smith, Jillian, author.
Title:	Taking control : a collection of inspiring stories for people living with multiple sclerosis / by Jillian Kingsford Smith.
ISBN:	9780987537508 (paperback)
Subjects:	Multiple sclerosis.
	Multiple sclerosis--Australia--Patients--Biography.
	Multiple sclerosis--Australia--Patients--Attitudes.
	Multiple sclerosis--Australia--Patients--Social conditions.
	Multiple sclerosis--Patients--Conduct of life.
	Multiple sclerosis--Patients--Services for.
	Multiple sclerosis--Patients--Life skills guides.
Dewey Number:	616.834006

Cover Design: Vanessa Maynard.

DEDICATION

To my family, who never stopped believing.

CONTENTS

FOREWORD

"The diagnosis is multiple sclerosis."
Being told you have MS is a life changer.

....

Jillian and I met a year ago through my role as the MS Nurse at Royal Brisbane and Women's Hospital in Queensland, Australia. Over the past 20 years I have come to know and been inspired by hundreds of people living with multiple sclerosis and their family and friends who share the journey.

An MS Nurse is one of the first health professionals on the scene and the one with whom an important nurse-patient relationship is established, often lasting for many years. Being an MS Nurse is a privilege, rich and rewarding, sharing times of sadness and also times of gladness – being part of our patients lives is where we want to be.

MS is most commonly diagnosed when people are 20 to 40 years of age: when life is already busy and complex - in the midst of university studies, beginning careers, establishing relationships, starting a family, managing hectic work places, juggling work and home responsibilities and busy with life's daily routines.

The news is initially overwhelming and it is not until a few weeks after diagnosis - often longer - that the reality of having MS sinks in and a myriad of questions about MS come to the fore. It is a steep learning curve in the early days.

Some of the common questions include: what causes MS, will the children get MS, queries on employment, who should be told about the diagnosis, what is a relapse, who to contact for advice when something new happens, what about travelling with MS medications, is it necessary to move house, what about taking complementary medicines, is there a special MS exercise regime and diet?

Each person has a different set of priorities and moves along this road at their own pace. It is very true that no two people experience MS in exactly the same way; every person is unique and the future course of their MS is unknown.

Learning to live with MS does take time. There are challenges and frustrations but also opportunities and achievements. Many people declutter their lives of the unnecessary stress and focus on the things that matter to them.

What a great idea to put together these 20 stories of people with MS in a book so that we can learn more and understand what it means to live with MS. Each story is unique, with a real and heartfelt personal account of living with MS, the ups and downs, the losses and the achievements, the hope, the grief and the joy.

The cure for MS has not yet been found but there are many researchers in Australia and also internationally searching for the cause of MS - and a cure.

Read these stories, enjoy, learn and be inspired.

Thank you Jillian and friends!

Kaye Hooper RN MPH
MS Nurse Consultant RBWH

MS Nurses work in MS Clinics and MS Societies around Australia and are committed to caring for and supporting people with MS.

- MS Nurses Australasia:
  www.msnainc.com.au
- International Organization of MS Nurses:
  www.iomsn.org

Find out more about MS and support the search for a cure.

About Kaye Hooper:

For the past 18 years Kaye has worked in the field of multiple sclerosis, providing integrated clinical health care for people with multiple sclerosis, managing the day to day running of MS clinics and engaging in research on multiple sclerosis.

She is a founding Board member of the International Organization of MS Nurses and founding President of MS Nurses Australasia as well as being an editorial board member of international journals and professional publications. She has co-authored an encyclopaedia of Multiple Sclerosis and authored articles and booklets on multiple sclerosis for the National Multiple Sclerosis Society (NMSS) in America.

INTRODUCTION

For many months this book was titled 'Losing Control.' The name came about because every single person I interviewed expressed at some point that they felt a loss of control over their life at the news of their diagnosis. You'll still see many of their quotes open each of the chapters.

It wasn't until I saw the initial cover designs for the book and actually saw the words 'Losing Control' in big type that I knew I had it inherently wrong. The stories of everyone in this book are about the exact opposite. They are about taking control.

I started developing this book about six weeks after my own diagnosis of MS. I couldn't find any material that gave me the necessary information to form an action plan. I didn't want to join a support group. In fact I really didn't want to tell anyone at all that I was living with MS. If people knew I had MS they might think I was less capable. I'm not sure how I thought I was going to write a book about MS without telling anyone but these are the small details we discard when we're on a mission!

Throughout the course of nine months of interviewing people from around Australia I unearthed a legion of courageous people who had been dealt a bad set of cards but went on to reform their deck. These people universally introduced themselves to me by saying "I'm happy to share my story but there's nothing special about me," or "I cant imagine why anyone would find me interesting."

But they had a bravery I didn't possess in opening their lives up to a stranger and taking me on a journey through their life with MS.

Their stories are indeed interesting and insightful and also served as an informal therapy for me. Their experiences taught me I could get on top of things. I could take control.

This book has taken me on an amazing journey. In the first month of my diagnosis well meaning friends and family would send me news clips of well-known Australian identities who were also dealing with MS. These were people like Chrissy Amphlett, Tim Ferguson and Paul Pisasale. None of these people let their MS get in the way of their life-long dreams. And they may even argue that living with MS made them all the more determined to succeed not in spite of the MS but because of it. I feel really blessed to have dealt with these three wonderful people while writing 'Taking Control' and their grace and guts to just 'get on with things' while living with MS has absolutely shaped my own response.

But I have been just as inspired and moved by the stories of the other, everyday people you'll meet in this book. They shared their stories of trying to conceive children and raise families, build a successful career, maintain a marriage or relationship, overcome depression, build businesses and chase their dreams - all while living with MS. Just like you, they have had good days and bad - and they very openly share those details. You will be moved by their own stories because you'll be able to relate. And in relating, you'll be able to take comfort that life does go on while living with MS. And maybe - just as it has for everyone in this book - it turns into something even better than what you had before.

JILLIAN KINGSFORD SMITH

"MS is scary. It's hard work and it forces you to make decisions you never thought you'd have to make. But I was finally starting to take control of this journey."

....

What you have to understand is that my life was a bit busy. I owned a successful digital marketing agency which kept me fully occupied, but on top of that I was dealing with a fairly messy separation from my husband, who'd left his life and mine in a fair mess. I was selling my house, trying to pack, get refinanced to buy a new house, attending business functions several times a week, sitting on the board of a local festival & then on top of that, dealing with my dog's phantom pregnancy.

Yes, life was quite full and chaotic and never shy of drama. But isn't every woman's life like that?

Which is why, when I finally presented to hospital, I found the look of disbelief on the doctor's faces hard to understand when they would ask me "why didn't you come in earlier?"

"Because I've been a bit busy and thought it would all just go away."

Their look told me I was absolutely crazy and I'm sure at that point they were making arrangements to transfer me to the psych ward, not neurology. What was about to happen over the next 30 days was nothing short of surreal for me and was the start of my 'busy life' being a very different one.

My saga starts when I woke up one morning feeling a bit shattered.

This was a fairly regular occurrence for me. I was suffering an enormous amount of anxiety on a daily basis about getting enough work done to service clients, trying to sort out the travesties of my soon to be ex-husband and just trying to stay ahead in the game of life in general. At that time I remember feeling so wiped out that the simple thought of just lying on the sofa all day sounded like bliss. Better than winning the lottery in fact.

I compromised by making a latte and plonking myself in front of the previous night's episode of "Real Housewives" before tackling the day.

Right away I noticed that the top of my left hand had no sensation. I tried tapping it with the fingers on my right hand but felt nothing. Weird...

My mobile phone rings, bringing the first client drama of the day. My niche is social media and I regularly have clients experiencing a Facebook drama that if you listened to them explain it, you'd think the world was coming to an end. No sooner do I sort that call out and the soon-to-be-ex-husband calls, raging about his own drama of the day. These calls usually went one of two ways: If he was bored, he'd call to check on the dog and talk about meaningless crap. If he felt stressed he would call to pick a fight. These were unpleasant, unnecessary and increasingly common. I'd usually remain calm until the last three minutes of the call, when I couldn't help myself any longer and would yell a volley of abuse down the line and hang up. Then I'd just be angry at myself for letting him get to me.

So by the time I was pulling up at my office that morning I felt exhausted. As I locked the car, I felt like I was getting the flu. I walked into my lobby and my receptionist cheerfully called hello and said how tired I looked. Yeah... Thanks...

Climbing two flights of stairs to my office seemed evil that day. 'Wow,' I thought. 'This flu is really bringing on the body aches and pains thick and fast.' I instantly dismissed everything as soon as I got into my office. I didn't have time to be sick.

By the middle of the day my 'flu' had gotten to a point where

I couldn't handle it any more. The headaches where muggy and horrendous and my body was aching. I went home with the thought of swallowing a few cold tablets and taking a nana nap. Hopefully a small rest would allow me to feel well enough to keep working through the night instead.

My nana nap turned into an all-nighter. I woke up early the next morning, still clothed and the television blaring. Coaxing myself to get mobile, I pep-talked myself into getting ready for a 9am appointment in the city.

While I was showering, I realized all the pep talking in the world couldn't cover up that I felt dreadful. I kept loosing balance in the shower. I dropped shampoo bottles and my hands wouldn't work in synchronicity to wash my hair.

'Phew,' I thought. 'This year's strain of flu must be bad; I really don't have time for this....'

I caught a bus into town and tried to pull myself together. I was pitching to a prestigious financial firm and I really wanted their business. I'm pretty comfortable pitching for business and talking with people in general. I figure if you know what you're talking about and have the confidence in your ability then you don't actually go in selling. You go in to have a conversation and try to solve people's problems.

I've pitched my company thousands of times over the last three years and I generally know every problem that needs a solution and every question that a potential client will ask to alleviate their fear of using social media. But this morning it felt like a nightmare keeping up with the conversation. I couldn't think one step ahead as usual. In fact, I could barely remember the words as they came out of this client's mouth. How I made it through an hour of conversation I have no idea.

When the meeting was finished, I remember standing up to shake hands but having to grab hold of my chair to steady myself.

"Whoa Jillian," laughed my client. "You weren't joking about this flu. It's really getting the better of you!"

I laughed it off but was secretly a bit surprised. This didn't feel good. I tentatively walked towards the elevators and when I was sure I was out of sight of everyone, started using the walls to prop myself up.

Quite by coincidence, a naturopath I was doing some work for had called while I was in the meeting. I returned her call and also told her about my symptoms. I described it as feeling off balance and tired, but with no coughing or congestion. She suggested I might even have a middle ear infection rather than the flu and that consulting an osteopath or chiropractor might be wise in case there was something wrong with my neck.

My neck did in fact feel quite stiff. But with the stress and anxiety I'd be enduring that was fairly normal. I knew I had a doctor's appointment at the end of the week anyway, so in the meantime I called a nearby chiropractic practice that was owned by an old school friend. They could see me that afternoon.

The chiropractor listened to my symptoms and did a preliminary exam. He wanted to take a quick X-ray as well just to be certain of what he was looking at. During the X-ray I had to stand very straight and still while I was having the images taken but all of a sudden I felt very dizzy and fainted. My chiropractor helped me come to while he was waiting for the films. We decided the best course of action was to rest for the remainder of the day and return the next day for a follow up.

By this stage I was clinging to the walls to walk and the world felt like it was tilting. Something felt seriously wrong but in my mind it was just sheer exhaustion. I had finally pushed myself to the limit and found that tipping point.

I returned to my chiropractor the next day and was still visibly off balance. He took one look at me and urged me to go straight to my doctor.

"I'm not going to treat you Jillian," he explained. "This is clearly something more serious and it would be remiss of me to treat you further until you've ruled out any neurological issues."

By that afternoon I was seeing my GP who concurred something quite serious was happening and she packed me straight off to the hospital; she didn't even wait for a referral to a neurologist.

So I found myself in the ER of Royal Brisbane & Women's Hospital on a Friday night. Let me just say that for anyone considering getting their MS or other ailment diagnosed, a Friday night in the ER of a major city hospital is probably not your best bet. At best, the ER was a mad house. At worst it was downright frightening. Nothing makes you consider the state of our public health system like peak hour in an ER.

Thanks to a very well versed letter from my GP to the admissions desk and the fact that I literally collapsed at the door I was whisked through the madding crowds and straight into a bed.

Lucky me. I was tucked into the hospital's ER right on peak hour. Friday afternoon is when most of the ambulances arrive to drop off the patients that the nursing homes, palliative care units and psych facilities don't want to deal with over the weekend. I could see the ambulances rolling up one by one and the chaos & cacophony was deafening.

First on the agenda was for a young nurse, curiously called 'Lovely Dave' to fit me with a cannula. I figured with a name like 'Lovely Dave' he would be sweet and gentle with a needle. And while quite lovely, my veins got quite the work out, being gouged not once or twice but three times until he finally discovered the sweet spot that didn't entail going straight through my vein to the other side.

A series of residents and their supervisors visited over the next several hours, each one grabbing at me to perform pretty much the same tests as the previous one. The symptoms remained the same as the previous few days, but to me, they were getting a little worse by the hour. Stroke or TIA seemed to be the popular diagnosis. One registrar recited a laundry list of possibilities to me, most of which were cardio-related ailments. He finished that list with 'or it could be MS, but you're getting a bit old for that.'

The minute I heard MS I immediately thought 'not me.' I didn't really know what MS was, but I knew enough to know I didn't want it. Images of walking weirdly or being in a wheel chair or dribbling constantly or having to be fed with a spoon went through my mind. Now I was really scared.

The doctors all agreed I needed to have an MRI as soon as possible. Unfortunately, the public health system's definition of ASAP is very different to my own.

"We're going to admit you until we can get you in to have an MRI," explained my resident, Dr Weibil. "We just don't think you should go home and be by yourself at this point. We need to keep an eye on things."

"Sure," I said. "What time tomorrow can we do the MRI?"

"Um, well, we don't like to schedule MRIs over the weekend," said Dr Weibil. "We should be able to get you in next Tuesday. Wednesday at the latest."

"You want me to stay in hospital five days waiting for an MRI so you can work out what's wrong with me?"

"Welcome to the public health system Jillian," said Dr Weibil. He wasn't smiling when he said that.

Despite it being 9pm at night I called my GP and explained the situation. I was sure there was some mistake and she could just call the hospital and have them schedule me in quicker. Not a chance....

My sister had actually driven up from New South Wales that day to spend a weekend with me. She walked in just as a coke head tried to throttle one of the nurses. I was so relieved to have my sister there. I was starting to realise that whatever was going on might be a bit more serious than I originally thought. I knew I wanted someone else there for the support but also to take notes of what the doctors were saying and doing in case I missed something - although I could see the concern in her eyes when ever a physical test was performed. She was starting to see that something wasn't right either.

At about 10pm I urged Rachel to go back to my place; there was little else she could do. She was exhausted from her drive and nobody had any clear idea as to when I'd be transferred to the DEM (Department of Emergency Medicine) ward. At about midnight Lovely Dave came back to see me. "You don't belong here love. It's only about to get crazier and you don't need to see this." He unlatched the brake on my bed and started wheeling me away. "We've got a couple of beds at the back of the ER ward that we're not meant to use because of the cut backs but I'm parking you down there so you can get some sleep."

He was right. The ER was littered with bloodied bodies, frantic paramedics dropping off and restocking, and the city's most hopeless citizens screeching, crying and vomiting. Whoever said Brisbane is just like a big country town hasn't experienced the hospital on a Friday night. I might as well have been in Sydney's Kings Cross.

A quiet bed tucked away from the mayhem brought a little bit of peace, but it also brought time to think. What the heck was going on? A few days ago I was running around, seeing clients and planning the next fabulous stage of my life. Now I was having conversations with medicos that involved words like stroke, TIA and multiple sclerosis. I was lying in a dark room by myself and I was scared. My often-prevailing positive attitude was finding it hard to poke through this one.

At about 6am I was finally transferred upstairs to the seventh floor. 'DEM' sounds exotic. It's a word that rolls off the tongue and emergency medicine implies a feeling of dynamic people rushing around solving medical mysteries. In reality it is a holding place for the people not easily slotted into any medical speciality. I was part of the melting pot now.

By mid morning I was wheeled down to have an MRI. I came to find out months later that one of the resident doctors, Dr Weibel, had fought to get me in for a sacred weekend MRI. It's just something they never do and this guy, whom I barely knew, had fought to get me into the system and diagnosed as quickly as possible. I will be forever grateful to him. I now hear stories about people waiting months to have their MS diagnosed due to a long wait on the diagnostic scans.

Within hours the results were back. Dr Weibel came up to my ward and announced that the MRI showed I had several brain lesions indicating multiple sclerosis. I asked exactly what that meant and he started describing how MS is a disease of the central nervous system or a process that involves an inflammatory demyelinating condition that causes lesions on the brain. I don't know why, but I pulled out my iPad and asked him to explain how the central nervous system worked and to spell words like demyelination. I think I was in shell shock. Dr Weibel left me in my bed alone for a while to think. He had more tests organised for me throughout that day and also explained I'd be transferred to the neurology ward.

I lay there trying not to cry. "Be strong. Be strong. Be strong," I kept chanting to myself. I couldn't really allow myself to think about anything other than what I was chanting otherwise I knew I'd break down.

An orderly arrived to wheel me off for a chest ultrasound at the same time that my parents walked in. My sister had called them and told them they should come to Brisbane. They live about five hours away in rural north-west New South Wales. The minute I saw Dad I just lost control. I burst into hysterical tears and clung to him. Through the tears I told him what Dr Weibel had said and thrust a Postit note into his hands with the doctor's mobile number. "Call him and get him to come back and explain everything."

In the ensuing days my family and I sat around in hospital waiting rooms feeling hollow. I don't think any of us knew how to process the diagnosis and it didn't help that there wasn't a lot of information we could be told. I think that's the most frustrating thing about MS. There's not a great deal of information that you can get your hands on so you can form an action plan. My family is all about problem solving and action plans. We're very decisive people so not being able to work on a five step plan was infuriating.

I spent that first night after the early and unconfirmed diagnosis Googling MS. There were a million entries about the topic but nothing that gave me what I was looking for. I was looking for someone to give me 'the plan.' I wanted it laid out for me. I wanted to find a document that said first do this, then do that and you'll feel like this. I was in a building surrounded by very smart people and had the power of the internet in my hands; still no one could tell me a damn thing.

The next few days were spent being wheeled in and out of various scans and tests. Literally every inch and organ in my body was examined in some way. I was still lodged in the Emergency Medicine wing until a bed in Neurology opened up. I had been moved from room to room for some reason. Each time I seemed to get closer to the losing ticket in the chook raffle. I was the youngest person by an easy 30 years and most definitely the only female. I thought the ER was scary but DEM was just surreal. My first room had an older man who leered at me through one eye while watching 'Tron' out the other. It blared from his ceiling mounted TV as he slouched in a recliner - hospital gown not working for his modesty at all. My next room afforded me a roommate who had a strange array of people pretending to be cab drivers walking in throughout the night, asking for 'Cyril' even though his name was Paul. I think he was a drug dealer. Finally, on my fifth day, I was transferred to an all female room. Mum and Dad were still in Brisbane and I could see their contempt for the situation. I had never stayed in hospital before and didn't know what was normal and what was unacceptable.

My roommates were Gloria, whose passion in life was genealogy. She immediately spied my surname and we had great conversations about my heritage. I became very fond of Gloria. Across from me was Elizabeth. Elizabeth didn't stay with us for too long. After spending 24 hours in our shared room it was found she was the source of an MRSA outbreak. Our room had to be literally hosed down, bedding destroyed and we were all rigorously screened. The ER was suddenly looking good again! Our third roommate was Catherine. Catherine kept to herself for the first day and mostly slept, until the drugs wore off and then she became very agitated. She was a pro at navigating the hospital system and it became obvious she belonged in the psych ward. While placid during the day, she would rant and rave at night. She would recant quite extravagant tales of betrayal and conspiracy. Very loudly. At 2am. Over the coming days she became more and more erratic. Psychiatrists would come and visit with her but she knew the system and was spectacularly adept at knowing the magic words to say to avoid being committed. Our MRSA lady was replaced with a dear old lady who had a wicked sense of humour. I believe she was probably in hospital with dementia-related issues. Her son, a well-know business columnist for the local paper, would visit her every morning. One day, a few hours after one of these visits, this lady buzzed one of the nurses to her bedside.

"Yes love. What can I do for you?" the nurse enquired.

She thrust a scrap of paper into the nurse's hand.

"I need you to call my son on this number immediately and tell him to come to the hospital and identify my body in the morgue."

"Love!" exclaimed the nurse. "Why would I do that? That's a horrible thing to say."

"Well I figure it's the only way I'm going to get my son up to the hospital to visit me."

And so went my days, nearly three weeks in fact, in the playground of Royal Brisbane Hospital.

My neurologist and the professor who became interested in my case were sure I had MS but it wasn't until the results of a lumbar puncture were back that they started having serious talks to me. They put me on an infusion of steroids over three days and started bringing a range of other specialists to talk with me.

My symptoms still hadn't improved at all and if anything, I was actually finding it harder to walk on my own and my spatial awareness - or proprioception - was really wonky.

One night, shortly after being transferred into the neurology ward, I got a bit of a fright when the dinner tray came around. (And no, it wasn't because of the hospital food.) I went to pick up my knife and fork and couldn't grip the fork properly in my left hand. On top of that, trying to coordinate to have the knife and fork work together proved too much. I looked at mum and was really alarmed. She could see the panic in my face as I broke into tears. I felt like some of the simplest tasks were starting to become impossible. Already walking was difficult, thinking hurt my head and now eating was a new challenge. My worst fears were starting to be realised. Life would never be the same.

Probably what panicked me the most was still not having a clear sense of what was going on. I was surrounded by a host a medical professionals but no one had a plan of action for me. It was all 'wait and see' and lots of unfinished sentences.

I'm a self-confessed A-type personality and not having a clear action plan doesn't work for me. I didn't know what the treatment plan was. I didn't know how long I'd be in hospital. I didn't know what the future might hold.

That night Mum and I ended up telephoning one of the registrar doctors who'd been attending to me. I was still sniffling and sobbing and I pleaded with her for more information. That's one of the most frustrating things about MS. There is no clear information to impart. You can be told scientifically that MS is the immune system attacking the central nervous system but no one can say what will happen when and what can be expected of treatment. There are no time frames, no certainties; only a frustrating set of variables.

I passed the time by becoming a sort of crash test dummy for the med students. I'm not sure how it all started; perhaps that combination of being considered 'too old' for MS as well as the fact that I really did have a mixed bag of symptoms with a fairly sudden onset. The allure proved too much and after willingly playing along with the first set of residents in a game of 'guess the disease' I fast gained the reputation for being a willing and enthusiastic subject. Before I knew it the faculty professors were bringing groups of students around to take my history, prod and poke me and generally pontificate as to what was wrong. I actually found the process really helpful as it educated me as much as entertained. Before long I was throwing the occasional mystery symptom in just to confuse them. About forty percent guessed MS within the allotted eight minutes. The usual suspects of stroke and TIA were often thrown out there. There was never any completely weird ailments suggested but it became obvious that MS was not straight forward to diagnose.

I've read research that says 80% of medical cases can be diagnosed from a patient history alone. I gave a very thorough family and medical history, but in my mind, there's no way they could have diagnosed the MS without a MRI and lumbar puncture.

I became worried about when I could get back to my business and attending to the needs of my clients. My house had also gone under contract when I was first admitted to hospital and I was keen to finish packing and begin looking for a new place. I was too busy worrying about the stuff I needed to try and control without realizing I was in an uncontrollable situation.

So what did I do? Nothing. Because there's nothing to be done. And that's part of dealing with a chronic illness. Working out what you can control and what you can't. When to worry and when to save your energy. It's taken me a while (and I've had a few false starts) but I've moved towards working out what I can comfortably do and what won't fit for my lifestyle with the MS anymore. I haven't allowed myself to grieve the things that are going to be too difficult to do in the future. I've instead decided to use my energy working out what I do want to do. It's actually created some great opportunities.

Working ridiculous hours to pay an astronomical mortgage and overpriced lifestyle wasn't sustainable. I loved my work but I wasn't overly happy. It had been a long time since I had actually sat down and reflected on what was important and what I wanted out of life. After my diagnosis with MS I took quite a bit of time off. About 12 months in fact. I originally planned to take three months off and even during this time I stupidly took on more work and clients. I could barely think yet here I was pitching for new work. It was truly ridiculous. About ten weeks after being diagnosed with MS I was hit with another massive health scare (but that's a whole other book!). It literally set me back on my arse. Never once did I say or think 'why me?' I knew it was that divine tap on the shoulder I needed to reassess my life and priorities. I hadn't gotten the lesson the first time round. I thought I had. I lay in hospital making all sorts of deals with the devil but I hadn't truly committed to making the necessary changes. Not mentally anyway. I'm pretty good at talking the talk, but even I knew I wasn't mentally or emotionally committed to slowing down and prioritising my health.

One of the scariest things that a diagnosis of MS can present is the possibility of loss of mobility. For me, I had lost all sensation in my left arm, leg and parts of my shoulder and chest. In the first ten days of the initial 'attack' I was literally dragging my left leg to be able to walk. My neurologist explained that the largest of my collection of brain lesions was sitting - like a proud fifty cent piece - right across the transmitters in my brain that carry the message down to the receptors in the various limbs that tell them to move.

I'm not used to being cooped up or incapacitated and I'm naturally fairly independent. Despite my lack of mobility I was constantly getting up to go to the rest room, stretch or see what was going on. I would walk along gripping the walls of the ward or lurch from one fixed object to the next, hoping like dear hell I wouldn't fall!

I imagine this ticked the nurses off no end and it wasn't long before a physiotherapist was called to equip me with various waking devices.

I'll never forget that day. Two physios proudly wheeled in a glider, a walker and a wheel chair, happily proclaiming that they had procured the latest model wheel chair and wasn't I lucky, as they were in high demand.

Seeing the glider wheeled in sent me over the edge. The glider is one of those clumsily welded contraptions with wheels that allow you to stand upright, rest your forearms on armrests and walk - or glide - along. I'm guessing the clever inventor thought that by giving it a regal and swanlike name, the sting of using one would be removed.

I lay there thinking 'I'm 40 years old. I used to run 50 kilometres a week. I used to teach yoga, dammit. And now you think its okay for me to use one of these?'

I don't know exactly who my anger and disbelief was directed towards. I felt humiliated and incapacitated and hopeless.

So the routine of my physical rehabilitation started. I often find that moving the body a little stills the mind and for me physiotherapy was a blessing. I wanted to regain as much mobility as possible but also wanted to feel that sense that I was proactive towards getting myself out of this mess. Of course, the cute hospital physio Reuben was an added bonus!

Reuben visited every day and set me up with a variety of exercises and routines I could do in bed. He also held the Holy Grail to my escape from hospital. I was desperate to get out and get home. I wanted the comfort of my own surrounds and the love of my little dachshund Pippy. Reuben explained that once the team of hospital physios felt I had enough strength to manage rehab, I could be transferred over to that unit. It was painted as this magical kingdom, where I would play all day in the gym, probably with other cute physios, and it would be a fun, healing time and I would have more freedom. Once I was in the rehab unit, I knew my mobility and balance would return quickly, because I would work hard and diligently and ace the tests. Then I could be released and go home and continue on as an outpatient.

I pushed hard for a place at the rehab unit and finally the transfer order came. I packed my bags and was transported across in the hospital mini-bus. In hindsight, they probably should have done the transfer in the dead of the night to soften the blow, because on arrival my bubble was quickly burst.

The resident therapist who performed my admission exam was quite sceptical about my mobility and inferred I had a long road ahead. He took me off the crutches I had started using and put me back on the glider. He really felt I would have at least three weeks in rehab before I could be discharged. I knew in my heart I was stronger than that. There was to be no physio that afternoon; no more work until the next day. I was left in the ward to stare at the ceiling again.

Rehab units are not a happy or motivating place. I guess I hadn't factored in the enormity of the disabilities that others face in the unit. While I was there, most of the other in-mates were elderly, immobile and sadly also dealing with severe neurological incapacitation.

I was wheeled into the dining room on my first night in rehab and sat at a table with plastic plates and utensils while the other dinner guests were fitted with bibs. The food was soft so as not to require chewing. Dinner conversation was not a priority.

At 7.05pm I decided going to bed was my only coping mechanism. Hopefully a night of sleep would block out the disbelief that the magical kingdom of rehab was a hell hole.

I was roomed with a pleasant looking lady who didn't feel the need for conversation. After her daughter had finished visiting I thought 'great, they'll turn the television off now and I can get some sleep.' At midnight the TV was still blaring and the nurses walking up and down the ward seemed not to notice. I lay there hour after hour listening to infomercials, motoring shows and a devastating medical program about new born babies with brain haemorrhages.

At 1am I'd had enough. I buzzed the nurse and politely asked if it was possible to have the TV turned off. It appeared my roommate was asleep so I didn't feel like I was offending anyone. The nurse curtly told me that having the TV on all night was the only way to keep this patient quiet and perhaps I should take a sleeping tablet instead. Unbelievable.

In the dead of the night I felt hopeless. I felt defeated and I felt hysterical. I lay there plotting my escape.

On first light the next morning I got up, dressed, slung my bag over my shoulder and called a cab. As I started hobbling down the hallway on my crutches a nurse came running up to me.

"What do you think you're doing?"

"I'm going home," I simply said.

"You can't just get up and walk out. You're not well enough to go home."

"Listen here," I said. "There's not a lot I can control at the moment but one thing I can control is the amount of rest I get and my attitude to wanting to get on top of this. In less than 12 hours you've managed to take both of those away from me. This is not the place for me to heal."

And you know what that nurse said back to me? She said "You're being very ungrateful. There are people who would love to be getting the help you're getting here in rehab."

I couldn't believe what I was hearing. I kept on hobbling out to the awaiting taxi. In a way it was the first time I started taking charge and making a decision as to how I wanted to take this thing on. I wasn't going to be broken down. I wanted to keep my head high and remain positive. MS is scary. It's hard work and it forces you to make decisions you never thought you'd have to make. But I was finally starting to take control of this journey.

***

After my escape from hospital I spent a few days packing up my apartment. I use the term 'pack up' loosely because all I was really doing was throwing possessions randomly into boxes. An occupational therapist had visited me in hospital to talk about an appropriate living environment going forward. Stairs would no longer be a good idea; if the house had hallways I should ensure they were wide enough for a wheelchair. Even the taps couldn't escape the scrutiny of the therapist. I should ensure they were the 'flick' variety that didn't require me to grip them. Mum was with me during this consultation and I could see her mind whirring at a hundred miles an hour. She was concerned that her own home had three steps leading up to the front door and that she had a bath and shower I wouldn't be easily able to get in and out of. I swear to god she was mentally calling the builder to make modifications before the meeting was even finished.

My own apartment had finally gone under contract after eight long months on the market and the therapist actually pointed out that I was in a prime position to find a new apartment that would accommodate my potentially declining mobility. Suddenly everything I wanted in a dream apartment changed. I was no longer thinking about proximity to the river or architectural features. I was prioritising bathroom layouts and proximity to the local supermarket - just in case I lost my licence to drive. A session with an occupational therapist can be very confronting but it is a necessary evil. They are trained to find solutions and brainstorm ideas to make your life easier and liveable. I specifically didn't want to think about the 'what if' of declining in mobility but despite its heartache it was a worthwhile experience. I went into the purchase of my next property knowing it was a very good compromise between my old desires and future requirements. Looking back this was the first time I started getting my head around the concept that everything about MS was going to be a trade off and you can live an incredibly fabulous life if you master the strategy.

So with four million boxes sitting in storage I went home to live with my parents for a month on the family property in rural New South Wales. It was a welcome respite because after packing up my dream home in Brisbane I just wanted to place as much distance between it and myself as possible. It represented my 'old' life. Not just because of a broken marriage but more so because I knew it wasn't a place I could sustain any longer. It was a two storey loft conversion that had stairs up to the master bedroom and was far too big to maintain by myself. The mortgage on it was also out of control and I inherently knew that I needed to start minimising costs and planning for a more solid financial future. I didn't quite know what my earning capacity would be going forward but I knew I couldn't maintain the pace I'd been working. I truly believe you can do anything you set your mind to but I knew that MS was a game changer on the work front. While I was only some five or six weeks into my journey with MS I knew I wouldn't have the energy to continue running my business at the pace and volume it had been operating and frankly I don't know how anyone could have sustained that pace regardless.

I had a few false starts with this theory all the same. The time down on my parent's property was intended to allow me the rest and solitude I needed to recover and process everything that had happened. Instead I turned it into a remote office and kept taking calls for new business. I could barely think, let alone type and I got the impression my conversations sounded like word soup. I was clearly in denial. I had no sense for how long these symptoms would last but I wasn't about to admit to anybody that I was working at less than 100% capacity. Looking back it was very brave but also quite damaging to keep pushing myself the way I did - not only mentally and physically, but emotionally. It created more stress to layer on top of an already tapped out situation.

At the end of the month Mum, Dad and I all travelled back up to Brisbane to meet with my neurologist for the first time since my hospital escape. He wanted to review my MRI's again and start talking about treatment options. Dr Blum had a fabulous demeanour; one that didn't make us feel rushed or unable to ask questions. He started by showing us the MRI, which was the first time I'd seen all the lesions that littered my brain. I think it was a bit of an eye opener for everyone, actually seeing the little blighters that were causing all the damage.

In the week leading up to my neurology appointment I'd been sent out an information pack on one of the popular medications at the time. It was a beautifully presented pack full of brochures and DVDs and pictures of happy-shiny people telling me how much better their life was through taking a twice weekly injection. I really had no idea what I was doing or looking at and certainly didn't understand that there were a range of medications on the market. Dr Blum walked us through three other alternatives. He very patiently explained how each worked and the various side effects. Medication A would help me achieve one outcome but I may get a brain tumour. Medication B would be quite good to help with my mobility issues but there'd been some instances of people getting cancer while taking it. Funnily enough I started reconciling that I was happy to take the chance that I wouldn't get a brain tumour but the possibility of cancer was more than I could bear.

Nothing prepares you for these conversations and it's a lot of information to take on board. I'm grateful that Dr Blum really took his time explaining everything, allowing me to ask many questions and take notes. He presented three treatment options that day but urged me to go away for a month, think about the benefits and side effects and also do my own research. If there's one piece of advice I have for anyone newly diagnosed, it would be to ask for the same scenario. There are so many treatments out there now with new ones available every month. The side effects are many and varied and you should take your time considering what you can live with and how the delivery of these treatments fits into your own life. I found a website called Patients Like Me incredibly helpful in explaining how different people felt whilst taking the medication that had been suggested by Dr Blum. Hearing how other people managed their medications and also fared while taking them absolutely shaped my treatment decision.

In the end the treatment decision was taken from my hands anyway. Some ten weeks after being diagnosed with multiple sclerosis I found a lump in my breast. I had just moved into my new apartment and was adjusting the underwire in my bra when I felt something strange. It was a large, oval-shaped lump, quite close to the surface. I freaked out and did what everyone does. I jumped onto Google and searched for information on breast lumps. I quickly came to the conclusion that I had a fibroadenoma, which could be easily dealt with. I mean, I had just been told I had MS. There's no god on earth that would also inflict me with breast cancer too.

I saw my GP two days later and she sent me off to have a mammogram the next day. After my first scan I was asked to sit in the waiting room. The tech came out and asked me to come back in for another scan, explaining she didn't quite get the required image the first time. Then after another thirty minute wait the head radiologist came out and asked me to come in for an ultrasound.

"I'm not going to beat around the bush with you Jillian," she said. "What I'm seeing is breast cancer and we need to do an ultrasound and biopsy to determine how far it's spread and what we're dealing with."

To cut a long story short the next seven days became a blur of doctor's appointments and hospital visits as we planned for immediate surgery. I had a mastectomy followed by stage one of a reconstruction and 28 lymph nodes removed. I went through my days trying to be as clinical as possible and numb to the emotion I was feeling. It was the only way I knew to cope and I was trying to protect my family and friends from an inconceivable situation. I didn't have anything in my kit of tricks to prepare me for this other than to realise that crumbling wouldn't achieve anything.

Not once did I say or think 'why me?' I looked at the impossible combination of MS and breast cancer as a way of having the message I needed to learn hammered home. I needed to prioritise my health and well being from here on in. I clearly hadn't gotten the message the first time round to slow down and make some necessary changes in life to protect my health, so maybe being told I had breast cancer might work. It did.

At this point I wrote to all my clients and told them the truth. I told them that I was taking an indefinite break from their work so I could undergo surgery and treatment. I don't know what reaction I expected but I was actually surrounded by an amazing amount of support and understanding. I felt like I finally had permission to stop and relax this poor little taxed-out body.

I decided to treat the breast cancer as a huge inconvenience from the start. I didn't want to give it any more credit than that of an annoying visitor; one that could be dealt with and dispensed after the necessary surgeries and treatments. I wanted it out of my body as soon as possible so I could resume the task of dealing with the MS. In consultation with my growing team of specialists, we decided to hold off on any MS treatments until after the surgeries, chemotherapy and radio-therapy; effectively some twelve to eighteen months down the track.

I quickly worked out during this whole process that that there were things I could control and things I had to allow my medical team to take charge of. But those things I could control were vitally important. I decided to start investing in myself. It took a few false starts but I realised that I was worth the effort. I only wanted to eat organic food, eliminating as many toxins as possible from my life. I wanted to get the necessary mental and physical rest so as my body could repair and this meant not putting myself in stressful situations that inflamed my emotions or created anxiety. I committed to exercising every day, getting sunlight and just simplifying life in general. I don't know why it took getting MS and cancer to invoke such a change but I highly recommend making changes to improve your health before getting the drastic tap on the shoulder I did.

***

As I near the 1 year anniversary of my diagnosis I still struggle with the concept of what 'work' is to me now. I'm dead scared of going back and resurrecting my business. I associate the pace I was working with getting sick again. I still feel exceptionally tired too. I can work for about two hours at a time on a computer and then my brain literally wants to shut down. I find that if I sit up in a chair for too long I get very sore and achy and my MS headaches start to rear their ugly little heads. So the thought of doing a long day in the office is not a reality any longer.

My neurologist suspects I had probably been living with MS for about 18 months or so before my formal diagnosis, but I know that most of the more impairing symptoms I feel now were done by that nasty, fifty cent-sized brain lesion that landed me in hospital. My neurologist has explained that this particular lesion, the largest of the lot, is sitting squarely over all the receptors in my brain that communicate with the other parts of my body that I'm experiencing the main difficulties with.

Coming to terms with a chronic illness is tricky but my psychologist Anne describes it perfectly. On one end of the spectrum you have your normal, healthy, full-energy, go-getting self. That's the person you're pretty comfortable with because you've lived with yourself like that for a long time. You know the play book, you know how to deal with things as they arise, and your problem-solving techniques are synced to this persona.

On the other end of the spectrum is the MS self. This is the person who is confronted with the new challenges that chronic illness brings. These are not challenges you're used to having to deal with. Processing how a chronic illness fits into the scheme of things is not something we generally sit around contemplating. How to deal with an unhappy client, how to pay this month's mortgage, how to patch up a fight with a loved one, how to cram everything into our already over-scheduled day..... That's what we're used to dealing with.

Suddenly we have this other persona - the MS self - that has to deal with all these new experiences and information. And that person does work out how to problem solve this new and unique set of challenges.

But what Anne explained was that there's an un-navigated and bumpy road to keep travelling constantly between the two personas and that's what can make the ride a bit frustrating. I kept travelling between the 'regular' self, who could work 15 hour days, do a 5km run then go drinking wine with girlfriends until 2am and the MS self, who was experiencing difficulties with all the things the regular self could do with her eyes closed. It was incredibly difficult.

I'm told that over time the travelling between the two becomes less frequent and the distance shorter. I guess the mind and spirit starts adjusting to the new set of rules you start instituting and a new set of problem solving skills are cultivated.

All the same I continue to express my sheer frustration with the changes that MS has brought. I can't get my mind around the fact that I still feel too wiped out to resume full time work. I've worked diligently all my life to get to where I am and I'm not afraid of hard work but at this point, doing more than a few hours a day just seems impossible.

At a recent psych session we delved straight into the work issue and why I was having such a hard time giving myself permission to scale back or make the necessary adjustments. On this occasion I was seeing an onco-psychiatrist named Jane Turner whom I had been referred to. I arrived on my walking stick and she asked how I felt about being seen with it.

"Fine," I replied. "I actually don't have an issue and don't really think about it that much. If I need it, I'd rather use it and feel a little more secure. People seem to clear a wide berth around me when they see the stick, which is what I'm actually after."

"Yes, people seem very scared of people on sticks and in wheel chairs don't they?" discussed Jane. "They steer clear in case it's contagious."

I recounted the story of Hayley, one of the other women inter-viewed for this book, who was being wheeled around a shopping centre in a wheel chair during one of her MS episodes and was increasingly annoyed about the looks of pity and confusion people directed her way. In the end her Mum went into a pharmacy, bought a big, white bandage and wrapped Hayley's legs so as to give people something else to look at and thus conclude what was wrong with her. Being the largely invisible disease that MS is, people can't reconcile when a person looks young and healthy but still can't function at the level they'd like.

Jane burst out laughing and starting pointing a finger at me.

"Jillian, don't you see the parallel between Hayley's situation and yours? It's as if you're the idiot bystander looking at yourself and internally screaming 'what's wrong with you? You look fine so get up and work.' Can't you recognise what you've been through and allow yourself the time you need to recover and work out what you need your life to look like for you to survive?"

Jane went on to further explain that I was setting myself up for failure by pushing myself to go back into a role or capacity that

I simply couldn't handle anymore. I'm a boilerplate A-Type personality, so nothing less than perfection is good enough. I hate letting people down and I hate presenting sloppy work. MS doesn't operate in the same way. It rebels rather than excels at being pushed. A person with MS who pushes themself ends up in a heap. Jane knew that for me, putting out sub-standard work would be soul-destroying and that would lead to depression. In tandem, bringing on constant fatigue would just end up intensifying the symptoms, which would lead to greater sickness. It was a swirling around the drain pipe effect I simply wouldn't be able to withstand.

The thing is, I know all this stuff logically but putting it into effect is so much harder in reality. Her analogy served well though and I think it was a major turning point for me. I can understand how others with a disability feel and I can absolutely empathise, but I couldn't seem to show myself the same respect.

In times of adversity we can choose fear or faith. I personally mix a little of the two, but generally faith wins out. Whether it's faith in the doctors, faith in the people around us who offer support or hopefully faith in yourself that you're strong enough to deal with everything MS brings to the table. Logically I knew what I needed to do and the changes I wanted to make and I've since come to realise that I was the only person who seemed to be standing in the way.

I certainly don't have all the answers; I've only just embarked on this journey. But I do know I wouldn't change a thing about the last twelve months. There have been times of immense anguish but there have also been times of celebrating new beginnings. MS has forced me to pull my life apart and recreate it with the next forty years in mind. Very rarely do we get the chance to examine what works and what doesn't and even rarer are the inciting incidents we need to make any long-lasting changes. While living with MS may seem unfathomable to many, to me it has opened the door to embracing some fabulous opportunities and creating a life that is kinder and more sustainable.

The Things Have Helped Me

"When things aren't adding up, start subtracting."

Website - Patients Like Me: This is an excellent website for tracking your MS symptoms & treatments. The forums on this site are also excellent sources of information.

http://www.patientslikeme.com/

Book – "Overcoming Multiple Sclerosis" Professor George Jelinek's book helped me understand some of the science & medicine behind MS. The diet he advocates is easy to understand & has made a difference in my own health. I think it's an excellent starting point in assisting you in making some lifestyle & treatment decisions.

Give yourself time: If at all possible, take some time off to rest & heal after your initial diagnosis. The first 12 months after are a huge period of adjustment - physically, mentally & emotionally. Despite how it might feel, you didn't just get MS overnight and your body isn't just going to recover from MS overnight. I believe the exacerbations are the body's way of saying it needs time out.

Make notes: Carry a notebook everywhere. I found it really helpful to jot notes when talking to doctors (eg record medical terms, medications etc to research later) right through to just jotting things I wanted to remember.... whether it's a notebook or an iPhone app.... don't be afraid to make notes of things you want to remember. It's easier (and far kinder) than beating yourself up later for 'brain fog.'

Take control of your medical care: Never be afraid to ask a doctor or specialist to explain something a second time and tell them when you don't understand something. Ask them to spell words you are unfamiliar with. This is YOUR health and body so don't be afraid to be in charge. Never be afraid to get a second opinion.

Exercise – Move it or lose it: I'm a big believer that exercise is critical in maintaining a healthy mind & body but also in overcoming illness. As difficult as it may feel, I ensure that I get some form of exercise daily. Some days it's a walk around the block with my dog, other days I knock out an hour on an elliptical machine. It's important to find a form of exercise you can manage AND enjoy with your MS. I find a session in a pool is a great way of cooling down in the warmer months and I also do my physical therapy in a pool because it eliminates my fear of falling over. My physio also highly recommends using the Nintendo Wii Fit program and balance board – there's some great balance exercises and yoga stretches on the game.

Make Life Easier!

- Get groceries home delivered. I use an excellent home delivery service for my organic fruit & veg.

- Accept help when offered and ask for it when needed.

- It's okay to say 'no' when you want to conserve your energy (or sanity). Practice it!

- Dragon Voice Recognition software is great for dictating emails, documents etc on your computer.

TIM FERGUSON

*"It was too scary to acknowledge the symptoms and how
I was losing control of my body."*

....

*Tim Ferguson is a widely acclaimed comedian, writer and
producer. At the age of 19 he formed the Doug Anthony Allstars
with friends Paul McDermott and Richard Fidler. Over a decade
long period DAAS broke box office records on 9 world tours and
released various books, comics, artworks, live recordings and
Australia's biggest selling independent album, ICON.*

*Since the group's split in 1994 Tim has toured the world
performing stand-up and musical comedy, and co-written dozens
of live stage comedy shows and light entertainment programmes.
He is recognised as Australia's foremost teacher of screen comedy.*

***

I guess I've been living with MS for nearly thirty years, but then
the first ten years of that was spent in denial as to what I actually
had. I was about 19 and had only just started doing silly things with
the Doug Anthony All Stars when the initial symptoms started to
show. I went to see a GP who concurred that my eyes were a little bit
out of whack but still looked perfectly fine and sent me on my way.
That was the first time that I recall any symptoms and I didn't think
anything of it at the time. It wasn't until years later, when I finally
had an MRI, that the neurologist could correlate particular brain

lesions to the trouble I'd been having with my eyes.

I never talked to anyone about what was going on because I figured everyone had weird stuff going on in their bodies. It wasn't until about 1992, some ten years after those initial problems with my eyesight, that I woke up and discovered the left side of my body had no feeling and it wasn't cooperating with me. At first I thought I was having a stroke because it was on my left side, but my speech was unaffected so I figured it was just exhaustion and hard living. But all of a sudden I couldn't dance and that's when I thought 'Well that's a problem.' Our shows were high-energy and built around singing and some fairly outlandish dancing. I went to see another GP who made me take an ECG test and then sent me home to rest.

But this 'thing' kept happening again and again without warning and I realised that whatever was going on was a real thing. I didn't know what it was but I knew I had no control over it. And the longer it went on, the closer I got to realising I had to stop being an Allstar, which was very difficult to comprehend. By that time, the group was very successful and I felt I had a whole machine of people relying on me and then all of a sudden I had to blow the whistle, which was no fun.

I transitioned from the physically draining performance and touring work of the Doug Anthony All Stars but still kept doing a bit of television work. The exhaustion element was still there and I shouldn't have been surprised when one morning I woke up and everything was haywire again.

So off I went to another neurologist who insisted I have an MRI. Having an MRI is not claustrophobic at all. You just hop into a cigar shaped container that clangs and have pictures taken of your head...nothing to worry about...NOT. But the MRI finally gave me a conclusive diagnosis. I clearly remember going back to see this neurologist and he sternly said "Yes Tim, it's Multiple Sclerosis." And I had no idea what that was. All I knew was it was one of those scary conditions that would make people shrink back from you and shriek out of sheer nervousness. And in fact, I'm sure that as a comedian I'd made jokes about it. But it still sounded better than what I thought it was going to be. I thought I was going to be told that I would die. So a big round of applause for me. I was relieved in a ridiculous way. I thought to myself 'I can deal with this. I can deal with anything so long as I can keep breathing.' In true form I was thinking about the next joke and how I could make this funny. I knew that I could still do stuff that no one else could do.... I'd just have to do it in a different way.

So I kept working and did what everyone else generally does: Not tell a soul. I didn't want to read about it. I didn't want to investigate it. The only thing I remembered from the neurologist was 'It doesn't kill you,' which was the only thought I kept in my mind because it was too scary to acknowledge the other symptoms and how I was losing control of my body.

I kept it all to myself because I didn't want to be any trouble. A lot of males feel this way. Women can get their mind around the concept of allowing people to worry and help a lot better than men can and possibly men would live a lot longer if they learned the skill. But it was just something I didn't want to burden other people with - particularly given it was invisible - and after all, I seemed fine so why freak everybody out? I just had this crushing guilt over the whole thing and I'm Catholic so we're better at concealing the pain than anyone!

I had several other very close friends who were oblivious to the diagnosis for a long, long time. None of them knew because I just didn't want anybody to worry. There's no benefit in other people worrying. But it's also a bravery thing and I think it takes a lot of guts to stand up and talk about this thing and share a burden with others. And actually letting people help is even harder.

The walking stick is what other people define us by, it's not for us to define ourselves by... otherwise we'd probably just take to bed all day and drink warm lemonade.

The burden of not telling anyone else hadn't really occurred to me. As a kid, I'd gone to nine different schools so the idea of reinventing myself on a regular basis wasn't anything that scared me. And the thing with MS is that it's invisible; nobody really knows unless you're limping or carrying a big stick. And even when I was working in television, I wore an eye patch to stop my double vision and people thought I was just playing the role of a pirate that day. And then I had to start walking with a stick and it got to the point where I was getting sick of people asking me what the stick was for. Australians, unlike so many other cultures on the planet, tend to be social etiquette morons. I think it's because Australians have an egalitarian streak that means they can randomly stop you in the street and ask what your health issues are.

I started developing some very smart answers for when people asked 'what's wrong with your leg?'

I'd reply 'What's wrong with your hair?' or one of my favourites 'I got attacked by a great white shark. Didn't you read about it in the newspapers?' Although that backfired on me once because the guy quickly replied that it must have been a pretty small shark....

One day I was talking to a mate and I finally admitted to him how bloody hard it was to keep my diagnosis under wraps after 15 years of keeping it to myself. I was also worried about what would happen to my career if anyone found out.

My mate said "Look at it this way. Which is harder? Hiding it or telling people and then trying to put a strategy in place to deal with it?"

I wouldn't recommend or dissuade people from 'coming out'. It's different for everyone. Some people are in a position where it would be appropriate to divulge everything and for others it can be a silent disease with no apparent or outwardly obvious symptoms. You've got to work out for yourself, given where you are in life and what you do, whether you need people to know and understand what's going on because your symptoms are visible or whether you can manage without the public knowing because it's not obvious that anything's going on anyway.

You get tired of people doing what that ridiculous television and radio advertisement suggests and that's asking 'How ARRREEEEE youooooo?' The RUOK? Day promotion has really changed how people enquire about you. The word 'are' becomes long and drawn out and tinged with feigned concern. And when you reply and say 'I'm fine,' the person asking the question just nods and says 'mmmm.... really?' (possibly with one eyebrow raised) as if to confirm their suspicion that you're not really okay but at least they've asked.

I regularly have other men who live with MS come up to me and quietly say 'Well I'll tell you how I really am,' but you know they're being mum about it where others are concerned. Men keep it to themselves because they're men. The last thing any man wants is for someone to ask how their health is. We're supermen, so why would anything be wrong?

I think for women it may be easier because women are used to talking about their feelings and the imbalances in their life. Men like to act like they're the king of the jungle because we're, well...mad.

Women love to get together and have coffee and talk about what's wrong. But men don't and never will. Some might say it's because of gender training but it's not. It's because of our DNA. This possibly makes me a very uncooperative patient. I don't like going to doctors – especially neurologists. I get particularly frustrated that none of them really understand much about MS. There's nothing much they can tell us and I lose a bit of patience when I hear time after time 'Nobody's really sure, but...' when talking about the various symptoms and outcomes.

Never-the-less I take my thoroughly annoying treatment every day but my opinion is because there's nothing much they can do, I don't end up in front of doctors very often.

My wife and I have signals now.

There's an understanding we have between us in asking how I'm feeling. She's very good at picking up when the first response to asking 'How are you today?' will require a second asking of 'How are you really?' That's when I normally come clean and reply with a shake of the head and a moan of 'Not so good.'

Nothing really scares my wife. She's completely undaunted by the MS and copes inordinately well. I put it down to the fact that she's Canadian and from the mountains, where they breed very tough women-folk. She's always said that whatever is going to happen is just going to happen but for now... hey, let's just get on with living life.

The only thing I think that could be a little bit maddening for her is that I equivocate. I don't know whether it's a trait that's built into me naturally or whether it's part of the MS and not really wanting to waste time or brain power on menial decisions.

The other day at the airport, one of the airline ground crew was assisting us in getting to our gate.

"Would you like to take your own wheel chair to the gate or use one of ours?"

And I said what I always do when presented with a multiple choice question, "yes."

"Um... okay, but what do you want," asked the patient ground crew again.

"Well, whatever you want."

"Yes, but we're asking you."

"But I'm flipping that right back at you..." and on and on... That can be a bit frustrating for people. I wasn't trained to ask for what I want and I think again, as a man we're not cut out to make small inconsequential decisions and then particularly we hate asking for any help. I also think the MS renders you intolerant of caring about the small stuff.

MS symptoms can demand a period of adjustment. It's learning to surrender to the condition. The first time you need to do something like call an airline and tell them you are disabled is a huge step to surrendering some control.

I still remember the first time I did that. I remember thinking to myself 'Oh God! I'm one of them. I've labelled myself; I have owned it now.' But for about the first decade or so that I had MS I refused to get an MRI and didn't really want to see a neurologist. I just didn't want to know. I knew it was bad. I just didn't know how bad. But it kept coming and going and I thought I'll just keep ploughing on. I was only having exacerbations every six months and so it was easy enough to ignore most of the time because the symptoms were very light and almost impossible for others to notice.

For me it's an alignment thing. From the beginning my eyesight didn't want to align. Other than that I would also get some buzzing and ringing and tingling, but all in different parts of my body, so back then I just assumed that I was having too much fun.... being the international comedy rock star in the making that I was. It was only when my leg became wonky that the MS actually became apparent to people. It operates at about 70% and it's only from the knee down that my leg doesn't want to cooperate. Everything else works brilliantly. And because it was mostly invisible I thought I could deny that there was a problem. I can even sit at a meeting with my head buzzing or shake hands without feeling the hand I was shaking. Although sometimes you'd know when you shook hands too hard because you'd get that look from the recipient of the handshake and feel like you'd violated some social etiquette!

I say yes first and worry about the consequences later.

Denial was, in fact, useful because I just kept getting stuff done. I kept saying 'yes' to projects and started a lot of new things, so for quite a while, pretending that I didn't have MS wasn't causing problems. Even now I still take too much on, but I'd rather take on too much then be tip-toeing around the world. So when the chance to write another book or make a TV series and work on a movie comes up, I just say 'yep – I'll do that. I say yes first and worry about the consequences later.

I'd rather give something a go and fail trying than sit around wondering if it might work. Performing ten shows at the Comedy Festival is a fine example of this. Everyone said 'don't do it. You shouldn't be doing it.' People queried if I was capable or had the energy but I didn't think in those terms for a split second.

And if I was incapable I'd find out the hard way but at least I'd given it a go. That's not to say that after a few weeks of doing a live comedy show every night the wear and tear won't show but if I didn't try it, it would be like taking part of my DNA away.

Achieving new goals is an act of will like anything else and also a lot of pepping yourself up. I often have talks to myself and phrase everything as if I'm already doing it. It requires conjuring an absolute belief that you are there and doing it already rather than working out if you can do something and how you are going to do it. When it came to the Comedy Festival I spoke to myself saying 'of course you're there and doing the show and if I was going to go and watch a comedy act about MS of course I'd wanted to see you playing the lead.' Self-belief and self-delusion are much the same, so choose the one that works!

Anyone with a medical condition would be familiar with receiving unsolicited advice and cures. On a fairly regular basis I receive emails from people offering up miraculous treatments for my MS.

Just last week I wrote back to one thanking her for the information but explaining that I have relapsing-remitting MS, for which there is not scientific cure. I phrased a very polite but strongly worded request to not bother me with miraculous cures any further. The woman wrote back almost immediately repeating but now amplifying her miraculous cure. She really wanted to convince me that her cure had worked on people and that it was amazing. I find it curious that these soothsayers don't immediately tell you what the cure is or how much it will cost.

One thing I absolutely won't spend any time or consideration on is the potions that get pushed. I figure that if there was any validity in them - if they had any lasting effect on MS - then the big pharmaceutical companies would have would have bought the formula, tweaked it a little and would now be making squillions of dollars out of it. But they haven't so I have no interest in it.

And then there's the naturopaths and kinesiologists and reiki masters and the list goes on....My view of naturopaths is fairly common knowledge and it's possible that I'm not entirely fair to them. But it's just because naturopathic remedies and advice hasn't resonated with me. Perhaps I haven't met the right person before but the few I have met want to immediately prescribe various supplements. They seem to make random suggestions of drinking rosehip juice while avoiding bananas at all expense. I just can't get my mind around it.

There seems to be an evangelisation of natural therapies and the proponents of them have an all or nothing approach. If you believe in one then you must believe in them all. I just sit firmly in the school that natural therapists make their money from the additional sale of herbal remedies. While I might quite like the massage or acupuncture it's the pushing of the potions I don't trust.

I did, however, try shiatsu massage once. I was given a lovely poetic talk about looking after the various aspects of my life and trying to find balance and that all made sense. I remember being there but feeling like I didn't have time for it. Shiatsu massage was developed in Japan early in the 20th Century. Although influenced by Western medicine, it has its basis in traditional Chinese medicine and follows the same principles of energy and meridians as acupressure. The practitioner uses fingers, thumbs, elbows, knees and even feet in a combination of massage techniques, applying pressure to key points to influence and stimulate energy flow in the body.

Once the session finished I felt good but still felt like all I'd done was lie there for 60 minutes and wasted time. It wasn't until I was walking home that I realised I was walking faster and further than I had it quite some time. It clearly felt good and seemed to have worked but to be honest I've never tried it again. I'm just too busy and it's not always easy getting places. That's the thing with MS. It would be great to spend more time seeking out all these things but the simple act of getting around and scheduling things isn't always easy.

I once chatted with Sydney's top acupuncturist at a lunch and quizzed him on the efficacy of acupuncture as a cure for MS.

His answer to me was a quick fire "no."

"Acupuncture cannot fix MS. Nobody can yet fix MS," he explained.

"Can you make it easier for me to walk?" I asked.

"Probably not," he answered.

"But I recently had a shiatsu massage and that seemed to help," I said hopefully.

"Then have another one," he concluded.

And that pretty much sums it up. Different things will work for different people but if it brings some relief or pleasure or relaxation, then keep doing it!

The other element to all of these different treatments and remedies is that surrendering time to the process can be an admission that everything is not okay. It can be particularly difficult for men to surrender time to our wellbeing. I know that's an absolutely stupid thing to suggest, but it feels like losing time that I could spend in other ways. I know I should spend more time thinking about my health, but I won't.

Good old-fashioned nutrition is important however. We all know we should eat more vegetables but steak is just so tasty and bacon with maple syrup is heaven.... so it's figuring out the trade off to living in the real world or becoming a hippy. (By the way, hippies drive me nuts because I like living in the real world. My personal belief is that capitalism is the greatest democratising force on the planet. It's flawed and wicked but we still get to vote.)

I know I should have broccoli for breakfast but I just can't get obsessed by it. When you've got MS it's easy to become fixated with different kinds of remedies. They're just so available and in your face through the internet or your email inbox. Even if you're not on the lookout for alternative treatments they're presented to us all the time and sometimes even by the GPs and friends you'd like to trust. And though they may mean well it's easy to become consumed by a certain approach or mislead by another. And Googling for information can scare the pants off you if the treatment doesn't relate to you or isn't framed correctly. MS is too particular and individual. One of the first things I always say to anyone newly diagnosed is to stay away from Google. All you will get is misdirection, advice from charlatans and scary stories. Let's face it, nobody knows anything about MS but there are an awful lot of people out there who say they do.

And the media are no better. I saw headlines this week about Annette Funicello's death. The media proclaimed "Mouseketeer Dies of MS!" But that's ridiculous. You can't die of MS. You can die from complications relating to MS but you can just as similarly die of complications due to stupidity. But no one ever blames stupidity for their death....

The vast majority of the people delivering information about MS – the media, the internet and even your friends – are wrong. It's important to work out what you can trust and what you'll ignore.

MS can come in like a tidal wave on people and so it can be really hard to find your way to do anything for a while. I don't know anyone with MS who hasn't changed their goals a little. We may even have to shorten the list of things we'd like to get done before God blows the whistle but it's not worth thinking about the things we can't do when you could instead spend your energy dreaming up the stuff that is doable. Or maybe even just a little bit beyond doable....

There's a great quote from one of the John le Carre characters in 'Smiley's People.' He says there's nothing as dangerous as a spy in a hurry and I sometimes think that people with MS can be like that. We're just at the point now that everyone is going to find themselves in eventually, but we've realised our clock really is ticking. Most people don't actually make that realisation until it's too late. And in that sense MS is a gift. I do things with MS that I would never have dreamed of and at a pace I would never have considered because everything matters to me now. We've just been told by nature that we haven't got a second to lose. I think it's why we're actually more productive too. Because this MS thing is so unpredictable and we don't know what's going to happen or when so there isn't a moment to waste.

I experience different mobility issues on different days and have a collection of sticks, walkers and wheelchairs depending on what's needed to get around. There's never been a time for me where I thought 'it's too hard to get around today. I just couldn't be bothered.' But there are times when my mobility challenges have to be taken into account. So I may just work from bed that day.

I never let the MS stop me but I might just have to put a bit more work into the logistics of the operation. As part of the 2013 Melbourne International Comedy Festival we reformed the Doug Anthony All Stars for one live show. Other than how we were going to perform the show itself I also had to work out how I was going to get onto the stage, move around the stage and then exit after the show. But it's all part of it. You can't let these challenges stop you from doing the things you love.

Energy levels are important to manage but I love working and if I'm with people and we're talking and working and banging our heads against the creative brick wall then really I can keep going for as long as I like. It's because the passion and drive is there. It seems to cut through anything else I might be feeling.

I remember a few years back I was on a film set and the budget was fairly tight. We had to keep shooting so as we could finish within one day. At that point we'd clocked up 21 hours on set and I was asked if I was alright.

"Well I have to be," I replied. "We just won't get this done if we don't keep pushing through." But I felt essentially okay because I was doing something I loved. My own particular energy levels don't suffer in that regard because I now make sure my days are largely filled with things I want to do. Generally if I'm doing something I love, something that's creative, I can keep going until they beg me to stop. Why waste time and energy otherwise?

I've heard the theory that MS affects a lot of people who seem to be the A-type personality. And to be honest, I've yet to meet a stupid person who has MS. They're usually very bright people, very-well read and interested in a diverse number of things but passionate about one or two things. So it might have something to do with having too many brain cells or too many synapses firing at once!

I guess we all work out different coping mechanisms and different ways to ignore 'it' – whatever the hell 'it' is. I also think the spirit of dynamism is important. You need to work out a way to adapt. And I think that necessity to adapt becomes very strong in people living with MS and so a lot of the time, that A-Type personality keeps shining through. We think more and plan more.

No one is going to stop me doing the things I want to do in life. Something else I've noticed about people who have lived with MS for a while is that they don't fear much anymore. They realise they've got bigger problems to deal with than worrying about their career or offending someone who gets in their way when they want or need to do something. My own priorities have absolutely changed. Gatekeepers are just going to have to deal with the fact that I'm in a hurry and they're in my god-damned way!

It might come across as sounding very glib to say 'chin up and just find a new life plan' but a great way to start is talking in the negative. By that I mean asking yourself things like 'what happens if I DONT start doing things I like?' or 'what would happen if I didn't plan to do anything today and instead chose to rest?' It could just mean that no matter how hard the MS is it might be the gift you needed to change your priorities.

Some people have asked me why I appear to be making fun of the condition in my show. But of course I'm going to make fun of it. The keys to comedy are anxiety and surprise. And if you've got MS, every single day begins with a little bit of anxiety as you awake to see the surprising symptoms that you will have. So it's already funny. It would be nice if people walked away from my show and thought about hugging the ones they love or being inspired to do something they always wanted to do but never got around to. But that's not really what my message is. It's about telling people whatever 'it' is, just get on with it.

My comedy show ends with me saying that people ask me how I am and the answer I give is the same answer everyone should give. It is "I'm getting on with it." Or if I'm feeling particularly feisty I might say "I'm getting on with it. What the fuck are you doing?" So people tend to walk away from my show liking the practicality of that. I think I'm saying that I'm not promising anything but I am getting on with it, albeit a bit slower than I used to. So whatever people have in front of them, it works as a good message. But people also say that it's inspiring to see me up on stage, despite the fact that I've got this thing and I reply to them "You, with that haircut, talk to me about having setbacks?"

Tim's Tips for Getting on With It

Be independent in trying to get ahead of the MS without relying solely on your neurologist. There's only so often you can hear a neurologist say "I don't know," at $200 an hour before you start realising that you need to play somewhat of a role in managing your own health.

**

How do I stay positive every day? I just remind myself that I've had breakfast today. It's a simple as that. When I know I've had breakfast it puts me miles ahead of the majority of the world's population. I call it 'comparative moralism.' Things could be much worse than just learning how to deal with MS every day.

**

If you have to surrender your licence at some point, don't panic. I've read that the average care costs about $5000 annually to keep on the road and that's already a lot of taxis. Most states in Australia will also provide discounted fares to people with disabilities.

**

The great thing is that society has as gone a long way to accommodate people with disabilities. Taxi companies have done a pretty good job of training their drivers in how to be familiar in dealing with people on sticks and in wheelchairs. You'll find they're very patient waiting for people to get in and out of cabs and just helpful in general because they realise that disabled people represent a fairly significant portion of their business.

**

I don't feel any responsibility to other people with MS any more than I would someone with, say, alopecia. I mean, everybody has something. But a small part of me hopes that others with MS see me still doing comedy and think 'well if he can do that, then anything's possible.' Or 'if he can still be funny then that does make anything is possible, because he doesn't look funny!'

**

I'm a big fan of Aristotle these days and he said 'There are thousands of ways to fail and only one way to succeed.' Now he didn't spell out what that one way was, but it's probably got something to do with hard work and persistence. And so however hard anything is for anybody, whatever it is we've chosen to do, we just have to approach it with hard work and persistence, as much as we can muster and that's what keeps me going.

HAYLEY DWYER

"My world was just turned upside down and I had lost control."

....

Waking up with the first symptoms of MS was just really strange. For me there weren't any physical symptoms, but rather sensations of disorientation and dizziness. To be honest, I felt very, very drunk! It was hard to stand up and the room was spinning; no matter whether I was lying down or sitting up I felt horrendously dizzy. When those feelings didn't subside I called my partner in.

"I feel drunk as a skunk," I joked to Drew. "What's going on? Did you hit me on the head during the night?" He was like 'no, no....!' But he sat with me for a bit until I came to the realization that I just couldn't go to work that day. As I went to get out of bed I nearly fell over. I couldn't tell which way was up or down or sideways.

Drew walked me into the bathroom to get changed but then instructed me to get back to bed once he realized how bad my sense of balance was. He rang my mum and she agreed she should come over and spend the day with me, just to be safe. But after 15 minutes with me she became very concerned.

"I'm taking you to the ER," said Mum. "This is not a middle ear infection; this is something serious. We're taking you straight to the emergency room."

"You don't think that's a bit of overkill Mum?" I said. "I'll just make an appointment with my GP."

Mum was insistent on taking me to the hospital though. She wanted someone to look at me straight away and do any of the required tests rather than getting a GP's referral to a specialist and then potentially waiting weeks for more appointments and tests.

To be honest I was starting to get a little worried myself. Once at the hospital, the emergency room doctors considered an aneurysm, a tumor, and even a stroke. CAT scans and MRIs were ordered. By this stage I knew something wasn't right. I was just hoping it's wasn't the worst kind of wrong.

Have you ever been to the doctor when you know there's nothing major wrong, but you're not really sure? You might find a lump on your arm and the doctor just confirms that you've been bitten by something, but it's not a tumor. I was pretty sure that would happen this time. That I was going to be told it was nothing major.

After a few more tests the head of neurology came to my bedside. He had both MRI results with him and started with the all-too-familiar tap, tap, tap, 'can you feel this vibration?' examination that I felt like I'd already done a hundred times.

"Yes, I'm afraid I'm confirming the diagnosis of MS," he said. I'll never forget the tone of his voice. I was thinking to myself 'what did you say? Are you serious?' Multiple Sclerosis hadn't even entered my mind, even though my grandmother has MS. Mum was with me and we both sat in silence for a minute.

By then my father and partner had also arrived. We couldn't do anything other than sit there and let the news sink in. We were all in shock. I just wanted to escape home, be in my own familiar surroundings and digest what I'd been told.

The neurologist explained that they were going to admit me to hospital and start the first of three rounds of IV steroids that would be administered daily. I stayed in hospital overnight but by the end of the second day I worked out that all I was doing was lying around, feeling dizzy and waiting for the next round of steroids. After the second treatment I announced to the nurses that I was going home. They were very opposed to me leaving but after a long and heated 'discussion' we all agreed that I would go home and come back the next day for my final round of treatment.

I already knew a little bit about the disease through my grandmother's experience. She was in her early 60s when she was diagnosed. She had balance issues and had tripped and broken the same foot three times before she was finally referred to a neurologist who confirmed she had MS. Mum told me she had been living with primary progressive MS for about fifteen years.

My doctors explained that I didn't have the same type of MS as my grandmother; that instead I had an episodic type or relapsing remitting. They handed me some literature to take home and read. And I guess between reading that and reflecting on my grandmother's situation I knew I didn't just wake up yesterday with MS; I'd had it for some time. After I read through the list of symptoms, I realized I'd been experiencing a lot of them in recent years. It also triggered a memory from four years previous when I was living in Melbourne. The soles of my feet went numb but I didn't even notice that it was happening until a friend commented that I was walking like a duck.

"Why are you walking funny?" she asked. "Are those shoes new?"

I realized that I couldn't actually feel the floor or my foot in the shoe, so my feet were flapping around as I walked. I saw a GP at the time, then a neurologist. The neurologist basically said to come back if it persisted for another week. And as it does with episodes it simply faded away and I didn't ever think about it again - until now. I recounted this experience to my current neurologist who was then able to diagnose that occurrence in Melbourne as my very first, official episode. It meant that I was able to go on a treatment for MS straight away, without having to wait for the next episode to strike again.

My mum is a nurse and I spent my first few weeks home from hospital at her place so she could help me a little if I needed it. Coincidentally on that first day home from hospital, the television ads from the MS Society started playing. They depict a person in a wheelchair, struggling to cut up an orange and feed himself.

To be honest I just broke down and lost it. Was this what life was going to be for me? Could a simple, everyday task of cutting an orange be my undoing? Was I about to subject my Mum to years of looking after her adult daughter?

I literally cried my way through a box of tissues believing all my dreams were shattered. All I could think was that I was never going to have kids; I was never going to get married because Drew wouldn't want me and my mum was going to have to bear the brunt of this. She'd have to feed me and cloth me. My world was just turned upside down and I had lost control.

But then reality kicked in. Hang on, I thought to myself. I was diagnosed three days ago but I didn't just get MS three days ago. I've had it pretty much all my life. I've been living okay so far and if someone asked me three days ago what my general health was like, I'd have to say I was pretty healthy. So I needed to adjust my outlook and realize that I was still pretty healthy, it's just that now I also happened to have MS.

The whole thing was still a huge adjustment but deep down I knew I could handle it. I thought the worst case scenario was I'd have a bad episode every four years or so where I might lose sensation or mobility in my leg, or my head might go a bit funny and I'd have to spend time in the hospital or time off work. I needed to be able to prepare for that and have a bit of a safety net for when those episodes might come.

I was ready to go back to work after about two weeks off. At the time, similar to my personal life, I didn't want anyone at work to know what had happened, mainly because there's a terrible misconception of MS out there. Even I had that misconception, despite the fact that my grandmother was living with MS, so really if anyone should have a better idea, it would be me; but if I was thinking the worst how could I expect my co-workers to think any differently?

Initially I only told my immediate managers about the diagnosis. Strangely I wasn't particularly worried about telling them – I just didn't want every single person at work knowing. MS was now a fact of life and if it all blew up for me and I got treated poorly, then I was just going to deal with that, because I couldn't avoid it.

My managers were absolutely fantastic though and have been extremely accommodating. We formulated some good solutions from the beginning that allow me to make up the hours when I'm feeling well or take a rest throughout the day if I need it. There's a first aid room at our offices if I ever need to lie down and I also purchased a car park in my building just in case. That was an added expense, but really worth it. Having said that, there's only really been about three occasions over the last few years where I've gone to lie down at work. If I'm feeling really bad I take annual leave so I can rest properly and get back on top of things.

The first treatment I tried after my diagnosis was Interferon injections and I would have more off days with those. I would go into work feeling like I had a flu. On those days, the fatigue was worse and I felt really tired, achy and grumpy and unfortunately I knew that lying down was the only thing that alleviated the symptoms.

My injections had to be taken every second day so I had arranged with my boss to come into work a bit later on the day after my injections. I found that if I could have a good sleep and get over the worst of the symptoms, then I could go to work and feel productive and more with it.

Over time, and as I became more comfortable with what I was dealing with, I started telling the people I had to work closely with.

One of the things I find I struggle with is my memory; it's shocking - really shocking. Especially when I'm tired or coming down with a cold or any kind of infection. In these situations I also struggle to find my words and I have to write everything down.

I remember explaining this to one of the girls I was working closely with on a big project. I asked her not to take offence if I asked her the same thing five times over a week. It was just that I hadn't written down what she'd said or I'd completely blanked on what we'd discussed. I asked her to be patient with me and she was fine.

If I hadn't explained about my MS I may have made things worse.

She now understood that I was actually listening to what she was saying and wasn't, in fact, an idiot! But by telling her up front she completely empathised. Bit by bit I've had more of those conversations with colleagues. I presume some of them told others and it's got around. They've now worked with me for several years and seen what having MS is like, so they don't have those horrific images of a helpless person in a wheel chair in their heads any longer.

The situation at work could have been very different though. I could have had a manager that wasn't prepared to be accommodating. They might have instead insisted I work within the same hours as everyone else. In the end I would have been under-productive and that would have annoyed the people around me, thus perpetuating the stigma of MS. But I'm really thankful that my company was so accommodating and all about finding a solution. Because of that I pull my weight and take tremendous pride in my work.

In those first few months after my diagnosis I found myself contemplating the stigma of MS in the workplace but also outside in the normal, everyday world. Simple situations would really bring home to me that people had no comprehension of what MS entails. It can largely be an invisible disease and I found this out the hard way when shortly after my first debilitating flare, my mum took me around the local shopping centre in a wheel chair. People would openly stare and try to figure out what was wrong with me. You could tell they were stumped because I wasn't slumped or withered and dribbling; I was simply feeling very dizzy. I looked like a healthy 30 year old but I was sitting in a wheel chair. It was so disconcerting that Mum found a pharmacy, bought a bright white bandage and wrapped it around my leg. People seemed to understand a leg injury and it stopped their staring.

Despite dealing with the stigma attached to MS head on and very quickly, I still have two big fears. I think anything else can happen to me, but I don't want to lose my eye sight. I've experienced an episode where I had some severe vision issues; but that was the only thing that went. I could still walk and think, but I couldn't see. When you're feeling fine and competent, but you just can't see properly, it's really frustrating. You can't read a book to pass the time, you can't watch TV, and you can't go to work. Basically you're left with your own thoughts.

During this particular episode where I lost my sight I was attempting to make a cup of tea by myself and misjudged where the tea cup was and poured boiling water all over my hands. After that incident I have so much more respect for fully functional blind people. I think sight is the worst sense to lose as it permeates every single aspect of your life. I can lose the movement of my legs; I can lose the sensation of touch; anything like that….but vision is just so integral to everything.

My second fear is that I won't be able to have the same interaction with my children that I would like to have. Statistically speaking, within a decade of being diagnosed fifty percent of people start developing secondary progressive MS, or SPMS. I don't have kids yet but I absolutely want to have them. I have a fear that it's going to be difficult for them and its going to be difficult for Drew, because he's going to have to take a considerably larger role then he would normally. I worry about the stress it might add to our relationship.

I want to be able to enjoy my child growing up while I still have good mobility. It's different when they become teenagers as I feel they'll be able to look after themselves more. If my mobility goes then, it's okay.

About two years into my diagnosis I decided to come off one type of treatment and try another. It's generally appropriate to allow for six months before starting a new treatment. My neurologist asked if I was considering having children and suggested that now would be a good time, while I was off the treatment, to try and fall pregnant.

I wasn't really ready to make that decision so quickly and I needed more time to weigh everything up, but she did instead suggest trying IVF treatments and freezing eggs at this point in my life so that even if I wasn't ready to have a child right now I still had some eggs that we could use at the appropriate point. I was advised that I should be off any MS medications for at least 6 months before even attempting to get pregnant. MS does not affect fertility, although certain MS treatments may have an effect on the development of the unborn baby. By taking the steps of IVF and freezing those eggs I can cease my treatment for 6 month and then have the eggs implanted immediately. We're at least reducing the risk that if it took a long time to fall pregnant naturally I'd be off my MS medication for that whole time.

Drew has actually blown my mind at how well he copes with the diagnosis. We had been together for two years before I was diagnosed. He owns two businesses and he doesn't stop ever. He has two phones and the laptop is permanently attached to him. He works a full day at one job and then comes home at night to run his other business. But the day after I was diagnosed and still in hospital for treatment he sat with me the entire day. All the phones were turned off and he just held my hand. He did nothing; he didn't even talk much, just held my hand. That's a big thing for him to do.

I remember he took me out to dinner the first night I was back at home. I had given our relationship a lot of thought whilst I was in the early days of my recovery. So I had this conversation all planned out in my mind.

I sat across the table from Drew and said "Look, I'm going to give you an out here, because I don't know exactly what this diagnosis means for me. And even worse, I don't know what it means for you. You didn't get into a relationship with someone with MS. You know a little bit more about what that entails now. I know I can't take on both my angst and yours so I'm giving you a free pass. You can go. I won't hold it against you, no hard feelings, I completely understand. I don't want you to stay with me because you feel bad," I explained.

Without even blinking, he reached across the table and grabbed my hand. He simply said "That will never, ever enter my mind."

So here I am four years down the track and the only thing that has changed in life is the way I perceive living it. It took some time but I decided not to get wrapped up in paranoia or fear and instead bring as much normalcy into my life as possible. I simply wanted to enjoy life. That's been the biggest change for me – the realization that I'm not going to be able to do everything forever. At some point it is guaranteed that my mobility will go downhill, whether it's because I'm dizzy constantly or I lose sensation in my leg. It's going to happen, so I'm trying to do everything I can, while I can. I'm not taking anything off the bucket list and I'm not turning down opportunities.

In a way I feel vindicated now that I know I have MS. I have an explanation as to why I become really tired when I get stressed. I now give myself permission to have a nap during the day if I feel the fatigue coming on, no questions asked! Before I'd say to myself 'suck it up, you're just feeling lazy.' But now I see the importance of treating myself better. I don't feel bad any more about saying no to activities that I know will knock me around for days afterwards.

It was maybe in the second year of my diagnosis that I told my neurologist that I was surprised she didn't send me for a new MRI. She said I could go and have one if I wanted but what would it ultimately prove?

"So what if you see another set of lesions in your brain?" she asked. "All that's going to do is stress you out and probably give you another attack. What really matters is what you're physically experiencing, not necessarily if spots are forming in your head."

And she's right. The reality of an MS diagnosis, as I have learnt through my own personal experience and through my friends with MS, is that it's very unlikely that an orange will be your undoing tomorrow. That your family will be there for you when you need them to walk slower or when you forget a dinner because you didn't put it in your calendar straight away or to give you a lift to a doctor's appointment when driving is not advisable because your vision is not up to scratch.

That rather than pity in a friend's eyes you will find admiration and respect that you manage do as much as you do with the limitations you have got, however minor or major, and still maintain the smile on your face....well, most days anyway!

Hayley's Tips for Living with MS

"I decided not to get wrapped up in paranoia or fear and instead bring as much normalcy into my life as possible."

If you're going to start treatment:

- Expect to be knocked around by the side effects to begin with.

- Make arrangements in advance to take responsibilities off your hands during the time you expect to experience any side effects. For instance ask someone else to do the school drop off in the morning and maybe take a half/whole day annual leave from work. It's important that you can just rest if you need to.

- If you don't experience any/too bad side effects then you'll get a pleasant surprise and be able to get on with life!

  P.S the needles (if that's the path you're going to take) are much quicker to get used to than you think!

Keep cool:

- Don't underestimate the effect that getting hot and bothered will have on your symptoms.

- Exercise in an air-conditioned gym, not outside in the summer time.

- Watch your internal temperature when exercising, not just the ambient temp. Learn your limits to how hot and sweaty you can allow yourself to become.

- If you don't have air-con installed at home then start saving for it. Government rebates are available and it can mean a good night's sleep and instant relief on a hot day.
- Have a good stash of movies or books for the time you will spend lying under the air-con at home in the middle of summer.

Working:

- If bladder control is a symptom and you work in a building with lifts prone to getting stuck (like mine), get into the habit of always going to the bathroom before you get into a lift!
- Be open and honest with your boss and the people who work closely with you about your MS and how you're feeling. They can be some of your best supporters of looking after yourself.

Rely on people who know:

- The MS Society is a great support network, with lots of resources and advice.
- Many city hospitals have specialised MS Clinics that are staffed with MS nurses who are very experienced and knowledgeable. For many of the day-to-day questions they are a great alternative to a private Neurologist.
- Remember that MS is different for every single person and there are no 'one size fits all' answers to your questions.

ALEXANDRA SMITH

*"Sometimes I can't stand the anxiety of how this game
is going to play out. I've always been a control freak
but one of the biggest things I battle is that I seem to have zero control
over what's going to happen."*

Pursuing a career as an army officer is understandably full of pressure. I started my military career at the Australian Defence Force Academy (ADFA) in Canberra training to become a commissioned officer. It's an intense four year programme, straight out of high school, that involves full-time study as well as undertaking field exercises. I had less university holidays and down time than most other kids my age and straight after completing the studies at ADFA I went on to the Royal Military College (RMC) Duntroon and the stress continued with incredibly difficult field exercises that put tremendous pressure on your body. Now that I look back, I'm convinced I had some early exacerbations of the MS during those field exercises. There were times my legs just wouldn't work properly and I couldn't explain it, but I know now it was my body demanding that I slow down. For twelve months we were under the pump. We worked six days a week, constantly being assessed. Our class started with 260 candidates and only 130 graduated. It's one of the hardest things I've ever done but I wouldn't change a thing.

After the high level of training I received from ADFA and RMC I was fairly accustomed to stress and pressure, but the level of fatigue

I was feeling for about a month before I was diagnosed with MS was uncharacteristic. I was falling asleep at my desk by 2pm every afternoon and also struggling to finish the mandatory PT (physical training) sessions, which for me was extremely unusual. As soon as I got home each evening I'd just want to go to bed. I kept saying to my partner Conrad "I'm just so tired. I really don't know what's going on." I was constantly exhausted no matter how much sleep I got at night.

I woke up on a Monday morning with some tingling and loss of sensation down one side of my body and a minor but intermittent paralysis. I was still walking around although I'd be dragging my leg to do it. I thought I'd slept on that side of my body weirdly and maybe pinched a nerve. I work with the medic team at my army base and mentioned it to them but they reckoned it would go away by the next day so I decided not to worry about it anymore. But the next day the loss of sensation had also spread into my right foot and I knew I should go to the RAP (regimental aid post) on their sick parade hours. Normally the doctors in this unit see a lot of common colds and pulled muscles so they really perked up when I presented with something different and everyone wanted to be involved!

A variety of theories were thrown around but it was my primary GP who suggested I may have a brain tumour and ordered a CT scan right away. Naturally I started panicking. My partner Conrad was working on a construction project and was unable to be contacted at the time but I remember calling him and leaving hysterical voice-mails about how the doctors thought I had a brain tumour and how I need him to be with me. By the time he listened to those messages the results were already back proving I didn't have a tumour.

The next track that the doctors went down was to suggest I had a migraine aura. Migraine auras accompany migraine attacks for about 20 – 30% of migraineurs. The most common aura symptoms are visual disturbances such as bright zigzag lines, flashing lights, difficulty in focusing or blind spots. Aura affects the visual field of both eyes despite often seeming to affect only one and lasts from five minutes to an hour before vision restores itself. Less commonly, aura affects sensation or speech and when several aura symptoms are present, they usually follow in succession.

I had suffered migraines before and knew the drill and the doctors agreed that the auras would go away within a few days. I went home to ride it out. However three days later there was still no change in my condition, except that the symptoms were no longer intermittent, they had become constant.

By this time I was quite concerned and turned to a good friend of mine, Katrina, who is an army doctor in another division. I called her for a second opinion and she wanted to see me immediately. She performed the same battery of neurological tests I'd already undergone and agreed that it could still be a migraine aura but that it could also be something else, such as multiple sclerosis or motor neurone disease. I immediately dismissed those suggestions as implausible but was referred to a neurologist for an emergency MRI, along with angiograms, EEGs & other neurological testing.

So here I was. Some seven days after waking up feeling 'weird' I was finally sitting in the waiting room of a neurologist awaiting the results. At that point I was still quite blasé about all the tests I had to gone through because I really didn't believe it was going to be anything serious. After all, I was young and healthy and had never had any major health issues. Unbeknownst to me, Conrad had been researching every neurological condition from A to Z.

That blasé mood was about to change. Conrad and I watched as my neurologist took the scans from me; left the office; walked back and forth, only popping her head out once to explain they were having 'computer issues.' When she was finally ready to talk to me I rose to walk into her office. "You should come too," she said to Conrad. Now I was really frightened.

"There are some abnormalities with your MRI," she said off the bat. "But we'll come back to that."

"No, no, no.... we won't come back to that," I said firmly. "Let's talk about that right now!"

"No Alex. I really want to go through your full medical history first so that we can be sure about my conclusions."

So I started all over again, explaining my symptoms from the onset – the paralysis, loss of movement, the headaches.

"Have you ever experienced this type of thing before?" she asked.

"Well actually, when I was in my first year of the army I'd wake up in the morning and my legs wouldn't move; my friends would have to help me get out of bed and take me to roll call. And in the years after that, I'd have days of dizziness where I couldn't even get out of bed. I thought that maybe I was just dehydrated. And even as far back as my university days I remember seeing a doctor because of numbness in my feet. That doctor just thought I was partying too hard so we all dismissed it."

"Okaaaayyyy....." she said. "I believe that was definitely the onset of your multiple sclerosis." With this she lit up the MRI scans and explained that I had lesions on my brain and spinal cord.

I burst into tears and Conrad reached over and held my hand.

"It's okay Al. We WILL get through this. I love you," he consoled me.

Then I blubbered to my neurologist "Can I still have kids?" She assured me I could and that the chance of them getting MS was not massively increased – maybe by just five percent. But I just cried. I couldn't focus on anything.

She then started a physical examination. Anyone who's been diagnosed with MS will know the standard tests. Can you feel hot and cold sensations? Can you feel the vibrating metal tool? How about this pin prick? Later I realised the severity of the situation really hit Conrad at this point. He could see the neurologist performing the tests but he could also see my lack of any reaction to the stimuli and I guess that must have been confronting.

I was admitted to hospital for a few days to undergo a steroid treatment before my scheduled Christmas/New Year leave. On my return I decided I would begin with the Copaxone treatment for MS.

My priority over the holiday break was to start telling my family and friends. To me it was important to control the flow of information; I didn't want anyone finding out that I had MS unless it was from me directly. It was a very surreal time and also very difficult dealing with the various reactions of everyone. I saw the full range of emotions from disbelief to sadness to concern.

My best friends had deployments in Afghanistan and Timor and the only way I could tell them was through email. I knew this wouldn't be the best way to break the news and I hated doing it, but the impact of them both finding out from someone else outweighed the improper etiquette.

The other tricky situation I had was how to break the news to my mother. Up until this point I hadn't wanted to worry her with what had been going on; at least not until I had a conclusive diagnosis to work with. I had organised for an aunt to fly from Melbourne to Sydney to be with my mother when I broke the news.

I called my mum the day my aunt arrived. "Oh my god. This is the best day of my life," exclaimed Mum when I telephoned. "You won't belief it but Donna surprised me with a visit today. The day can't get any better!"

"Actually Mum, I sent Donna to be with you. You don't know this but I've been having a lot of medical issues over the last few weeks." As I described what had been going on and the news the neurologist had given me, Mum became very defensive and demanded to know why she was the last one to find out. We talked through everything and she decided to come to be with me immediately. Her arrival coincided with the first day I started on the steroid treatment for MS.

My parent's reaction to the news was diverse but fairly normal. My dad is retired military, so his reaction was analytical and action-oriented. My mother wanted to know what treatment options were available, what was the best treatment, hospital and doctor and she was resolute on going to the ends of the earth to find the best solution.

The army's reaction was very supportive. I decided from the onset to be very up front with my commanding officers and people I work with. It was important to me that everyone understand the reason behind my eventual medical discharge from ROSO (Return of Service Obligations) wasn't a psych discharge and that I wasn't a 'linga' or malingerer. My theory is that the more people I tell, the more awareness there will be around MS.

Serving my country was all I'd ever wanted to do, but the decision to leave the army was pretty cut and dry. Once I had that diagnosis I knew immediately that I wasn't compatible with service anymore. I knew physically it would be impossible but also I knew I didn't want to be in a career where my disease limited me. I wouldn't be able to deploy or go into the field – I basically couldn't do anything that I wanted to do in the army any more.

Since my diagnosis I've had to organise the deployment of over a dozen people and it was a gut-wrenching experience. I knew that under different circumstance I would have been the first pick for these deployments. I couldn't handle having 'what might have been' thrown in my face.

What I continue to struggle with is that most of the officers I serve with cant understand why I'm being discharged. They know I have MS and I'm surrounded by people in the medical profession because I work in the army's medical office. They still see me as a capable person who performs her duties every day. My colleagues don't fully understand why having MS and deploying aren't compatible. I know that when I signed up I had to be medically fit, I had to pass all my Basic Fitness Assessments (BFAs) and be a certain mould of person. The person I was when I signed up and the person I am now are not the same.

While my life is in a state of limbo at the moment as I work out what I'm going to do with my career next, the army have been amazingly supportive during this process. They have extended themselves more than I could have imagined. They were very active in providing every resource to get a diagnosis and the eventual treatment of the MS and

I have been counselled and mentored through the various decisions I needed to make.

I've decided to look at my discharge as a new stage of my life that probably suits Conrad and I better anyway. While serving in the army had been fabulous, it had been difficult to establish a home base due to the various postings to new bases. Conrad now had the opportunity to enter the police force, which had been a lifelong dream of his and I was able to pursue a new career in nursing, which I'd become attracted to. We finally had the certainty of staying in one place long enough to complete study for our new careers.

The only question I asked my neurologist on the day I was diagnosed was whether I could eventually have children. She explained that having children was actually encouraged due to the positive effects that progesterone production can have on the brain.

There is no evidence that MS impairs fertility or congenital malformations. According to the National MS Society of America, several studies of large numbers of women have repeatedly demonstrated that pregnancy, labor, delivery and the incidence of foetal complications are no different in women who have MS than in control groups without the disease.

Before 1950, most women with MS were counselled to avoid pregnancy because of the belief that it might make their MS worse. Over the past 40 years, many studies have been undertaken on hundreds of women with MS, and they have almost all reached the opposite conclusion: that pregnancy reduces the number of MS exacerbations, especially in the second and third trimesters.

In general, pregnancy does not appear to affect the long-term clinical course of MS. Women who have MS and wish to have a family can usually do so successfully with the assistance of their neurologist and obstetrician.[1]

My biggest concern with having children at this point is whether I'd be passing the disease onto my children. I worry whether I'm being selfish by possibly giving them an incurable disease and whether I should cross my fingers that my children are boys and thus have less chance of manifesting MS. I know the chance of passing MS onto your children is around the 5 to 10% mark, but it's still a risk that needs to be calculated.

A 2006 study from the Mayo Clinic in Rochester MN, USA found that in a group of 441 children with a parent with multiple sclerosis, fathers with MS were more likely to pass on the disease to children than mothers with MS. Although MS is not directly hereditary, a person who has a first-degree relative (such as a parent or sibling) with MS has a greater risk of developing MS than a person with no MS in the family. Researchers believe that MS occurs in individuals who have genes that make them susceptible to an unknown environmental trigger or triggers. In addition, women are twice as likely as men to develop MS. The reason for this difference is unknown.[2]

When I was first diagnosed, I immediately confused the symptoms of MS with another chronic disease and thought my life was over. Now that I have a far better understanding of MS and have discounted much of the stigma attached to it

One of the worst moments I've experienced with my MS was at the hospital clinic during the first treatment of steroids. I was really nervous and the guy next to me started volunteering his life story and telling me how MS had ruined his life. He said he could no longer play sport or even walk up a hill without getting puffed.

I started to freak out because sport has always been a huge part of my life. It's my passion and my outlet. What was I going to do if I could no longer play sport? You have to remember that everything about MS was so new to me. I hadn't done a lot of research or talked to others. I didn't know what to expect and I was so nervous about everything. On top of that I couldn't think straight anyway!

Eventually one of the MS nurses came over to me. "Alex, you have to remember everyone's MS is different," she said. After this she had to go on a break but before she left she asked Conrad if he'd mind waiting outside because the clinic was getting very busy. What I didn't know at the time was that this nurse actually sat outside with Conrad for half an hour, counselling him to keep me positive and explaining that MS manifests itself in so many ways and that a patient's positivity played an enormous role.

That same day another patient offered the advice that I couldn't let MS beat me. I thought it was a strange thing to say at the time, but I've since come to realise that you can't let it rule your life. You have to find your own sense of balance in everything you do. There's plenty of people with varying degrees of advice and theories out there, but I've found that by adapting different techniques to suit me – be it diet or how to manage my time – I have developed a plan that works. I don't let the MS rule my life and I certainly won't let it beat me. I feel really lucky that I've found out at a young age that I have MS. I've been able to start my treatment early and I've got ten years on a lot of people who are only just getting treated now.

It's been 12 months since my diagnosis and I still can't bring myself to read too much about MS. I guess I'm burying my head in the sand, but there are just so many other things to get used to. My partner Conrad has done a tonne of research. I think it's how he copes with it. I still don't want to know too much; I can't handle it. I don't want to watch the people in motorised wheel chairs. It's too confronting.

One thing we have done is changed our diet totally. The research Conrad has read pointed to the fact that cutting out all gluten, dairy & sugar was beneficial for people with MS and other autoimmune diseases. The change the diet brought about was amazing and we've found it very easy to stick to because we feel so good. We also try to maintain our active lifestyles, getting to the gym throughout the week. I tend to go to the gym in the evening so as I can come home and go to bed afterwards.

For me it's been really important to work out who my key support group is. I can imagine that for many people living with MS, their support group may be made up of therapists or doctors or even a formal support group that caters to people with chronic illnesses, but for me I knew very quickly that my partner, close friends and immediate family where who I needed. What I need to remind my support group about all the time is that I don't need to talk about

MS constantly. I want to talk about what's going on in their life and what's important to them. It's not all about my illness.

Realising some of my own limitations now has been a huge thing for me to adjust to. I now know that my symptoms start as soon as I get fatigued and because of that, I have to rest a bit more often. But the army teaches us from the start to push through things; to endure more than most people would. I used to know exactly how far I could push my body because I've had over a decade of doing extreme training. I mean, we used to go up to nine days without sleep! But the MS brings its own set of rules and I haven't quite learned all the new regulations yet. No one in the army has ever been concerned when I've had to take time off, but the very act of asking for the time off has been very stressful for me. I felt that I was being judged or that people would think I was less capable. The logical part of your brain knows this isn't true, but the emotional part of you can't reconcile that.

I actually think the diagnosis has given me a new lease on life. I want to go out now and do things I've always dreamed of doing but had always put aside because of my commitment to a military career. I have a really positive outlook on my future prognosis but I still want to live life to its fullest while I can. Last week I booked a holiday to China. I've always wanted to climb the Great Wall of China and now I'm going to do it while I still can. I've re-prioritised what's important to me. While I'm forever grateful to the Army for the career and opportunities it's given me, my focus now is very much on my health and relationship with my partner.

Sometimes I can't stand the anxiety of how this game is going to play out. I've always been a control freak but one of the biggest things I battle is that I seem to have zero control over what's going to happen. I just have to let it happen however it's going to happen.

Alex's Tips for Living with MS

"Life is like a photograph, we develop from the negatives."

Humour: For me and my partner this has been a big part of our success in coping with the life-altering news. It helps us to breaks down the barriers, make light of the situation and calm the nerves. Not for everyone and not for all occasions, but humour has helped me more than I can express.

Communicating the news: You must come to terms with it before you can deal with others. You are the most important person in this equation. However a time will come when you start telling others. The hardest thing for me was telling others, because their reactions were often worse than mine. I came to terms with MS in my own time but I believe I did this quite quickly and then immediately channelled my thinking into ways to change my life to suit this new development. But every time I had to tell someone else, I relived the drama and emotional trauma of it. So don't be afraid to wait to tell people or utilize your close friends and family to tell others for you, so by the time you talk to them, they have had time to process. It's not easy to listen to your close relatives or friends become over-emotional and cry, swear or having a mini breakdown. It's not great for you recovery either, as this is about you, not about consoling others. My partner was a great support in this area, he would subtly tell people, so by the time I bought it up in conversation, they were a great support and had only positive things to say.

Diet: Short term pain, long term gain has never been truer. The gains that can be achieved from a healthy lifestyle are huge. We are talking possible increase in life expectancy and a better quality of life - surely worth the short term pain? A dietary guide I can recommend is 'Whole 30'. It is an extreme food plan to work all the crap out of your body, it is a Paleo-based diet and an excellent tool to demonstrate what you need and how delicious healthy eating is.

The information that impacted my life the most was:

• Dairy and gluten work as inflammatory agents in the body, and let's face it we don't need any inflammation than what is already on our brains; and

• Ginger is great for us, as it is a natural anti-inflammatory.

I was amazed how often MS was specifically mentioned in the Whole 30. The dietary guide gives you a good base to become healthy and to understand the effects of nutrition on your body. No one can prove that diet is the reason for reductions in episodes, but everyone that has changed their way of eating can tell you it has helped them.

Support and Rest: Allow the support and accept that you will change. In the defence force you are taught to push through the pain and the fatigue; I was taught how far my body can be pushed and I always felt that I needed to be strong and not show any weakness. Although you are encouraged to work as teams, I would still have felt it was a sign of weakness or incompetence to have to rest or ask someone else to complete something for me. I needed to alter that thought process and when I start to feel symptoms or fatigue I need to act on that and have 'me' time and rest. You cannot push through MS, you need to be aware of it.

Do it your way: Don't let people become overwhelming. There is a big difference between support and being overpowered. This is your disease and you have to cope with it your way. Only you know 'your MS.' It is different from everyone else's and what works for me, does not mean it will for you. So find your own ways to live with MS.

Keep Control: Do not let MS beat or control you. You must take control. You should try to control your MS - I do not mean control your symptoms or the disease - that is not possible. You need to control your attitude. You will be amazed at what a positive attitude can do for you.

Knowledge is key to maintaining control: There is so much information out there about MS so be careful where you source it! But don't stick your head in the sand. Be prepared for doctors appointments. I always have a list of questions for mine. It helps me cope a little better, as it brings structure and goals to my appointments and it helps me learn more about my MS.

Be Open Minded: Besides conventional medical advice and treatments, there also some alternative medicines or therapies that can be useful. Things such as traditional Chinese medicine (TCM), naturopathy and remedial massage are all fairly common these days. It's all about finding what works for you. A naturopath is where I learnt that swimming can be a tremendously beneficial exercise - low impact, but works both sides of the brain, so keeps you more active and alert. None of the doctors I spoke to ever gave me that information. Utilize all resources available.

REGAN TRASK

"I'm really happy with the person I've become since my diagnosis. I've had to learn to let go of the things that just aren't important. Living with MS makes you reconsider what really matters in life."

....

It would be easy for me to look at my diagnosis of MS as a curse. I mean, overnight I had to learn to contend with some of the physical and neurological challenges the illness presents; I had my life turned upside down when my long-term boyfriend decided he didn't want to deal with a girlfriend who had a chronic illness, and I also found myself with a healthy whack of depression. But on the flip side, if I hadn't discovered that I had MS, I might still be stuck in a rut with a man who wanted very different things in life to me, I would never have found out exactly how strong I am and I wouldn't be blessed with the amazing fiancé and son I now have.

I was diagnosed in May 2005 but the lead up to my diagnosis took a long time. For many months I had been having headaches and feeling dizzy and fatigued and just generally felt 'heavy' all over. On a number of occasions I went back to my GP, unhappy with n ot finding a reason for all these anomalies despite a clear CT scan and relatively normal blood work. It was only that I saw a different GP in the practice who referred me to an optometrist that I started to get somewhere. By then I was having cloudiness in the bottom right corner of my right eye and the optometrist I consulted referred me on to a neuro-opthamologist within the hour.

He carried out a number of tests and told me that it could be one of three things but he was confident it was MS - emphasising that MS was actually the 'best' option out of the three! He explained that if what I was experiencing was optic neuritis then it would progressively get worse over the coming days. He was spot on. I lost sight completely in the right eye within 48 hours and my left eye also had significant blurring. A couple of weeks later I had an MRI that confirmed the diagnosis of MS.

At the time I was working with Pfizer, a multinational pharmaceutical company. They were absolutely amazing in how they accommodated my diagnosis. They said to me "Just do what you can do. You have our support one hundred percent in whatever way you need it." In the early days after my diagnosis I tried a number of different treatments and none of them seemed to work for me. My neurologist suggested a 12 month protocol of chemotherapy as a way of resetting my immune system. It's a bit like a 'Control-Alt-Delete' mechanism for your body. I agreed to the treatment and during this time Pfizer went to the ends of the earth to prioritise my health and wellbeing. They ensured I had a job to return to, which eliminated any stress I felt about the future of my career. The company even redeveloped my position to incorporate a range of different responsibilities, any of which I could work towards depending on my energy levels and treatment schedule.

Only my manager knew of my condition. Pfizer really bent over backwards to assist me in my role and some of the newer girls thought management were displaying favouritism. These girls didn't know I had MS and really there was no reason to tell them. However, during one MS flare I went to work but needed to use my walking stick. Before going to work I decided to ask my manager to have a chat to the girls about why I'd be using a stick. I wanted to try and control the information and gossip before it got out of hand. They were already speculating about the preferred treatment I was receiving and frankly I was sick of hearing all the rubbish. After that little 'chat' the girls were awfully nice to me and started treating me differently and I had to pull them up.

"Don't pretend you like me now,' I said to the girls. "I don't want you to feel sorry for me. It's business as normal for me and that's why I'm here on a walking stick today. But I tell you what, perhaps in the future you'll stop and think that everyone has stuff going on in their lives and maybe one day you'll need someone to give you a bit of a break."

Unfortunately the general public aren't very clever when it comes to chronic illness. If we could wear a sign on our forehead that says "I have MS. You can't see it but that's why I might be a bit slow or aloof or trip or walk a little funny some times. I'm not drunk or stupid." I don't want anyone feeling sorry for me or thinking I'm less capable. Generally speaking I just want to get on with things. But when I was working I did need a little bit of extra help – whether I realised it or not – and I was lucky to have an employer who willingly provided that, and did so without fuss. It was just the younger girls (who really didn't have any point of reference for what I was going through) who became a little silly at times.

Pfizer were just fantastic in their approach to keep me working for the company. In the end, it was me who worried the attention I was getting wasn't fair to other employees and about two years after my diagnosis I resigned. Even then, the general manager kept trying to persuade me to stay on.

At first I wasn't really bothered by the innuendo or gossip going on in the workplace as to my days off or being able to manage my own schedule, but over time I've come to believe that controlling the information and message to the people you work with is a good strategy. Obviously each work situation is going to be different, but ultimately I think you need to decide a strategy of what you tell to whom. I found a good rule of thumb was to tell only those that my MS impacted. Make sure you're the one controlling the flow of information. I think if you're seen to be getting on with life, then everyone else has no choice but to also get on with things too. It makes for an environment that is a lot less stressful and easier to work in!

I chose to be up-front with my employers that I had MS. I've gone into every new employment situation believing honesty was the best policy and that if they didn't want to employ me because I was living with MS, then I didn't want to work with that company. I don't necessarily go and tell everyone on the team I work with, just the person employing me is all that really matters to me. It's not something I'm excited to share with anybody, but if I need to I will. You would hope that by telling your managers you could then work together to find a solution to any employment issues that may arise because of the MS. For me, I need one day a month away from work to get my treatment. With any new job I needed to know that a leave request would be accommodated. In my previous full time roles I was able to come and go as I needed all the time, so long as I achieved the outcomes that had been set for me each month. Now I work part time and I'm able to schedule my treatment for the days I don't work.

I've come across people with MS who have already given up early in the game. There's one woman at my treatment centre who is still walking fine but the first time I met her she proudly told me that she'd already bought a mobility scooter. I just see that as giving up. I think your mind and willpower are very strong things but if you've gone from walking to the mobility scooter without knowing what the time in between might hold then you've allowed yourself to believe that the future is all downhill.

I was so embarrassed for a long time that I was taking medication for depression but then I realised the tablets help me get through the tough times that MS can bring.

I suffered from depression after my diagnosis. I had an anxiety attack after my first steroid treatment & I was 100% convinced I was dying. The doctors tried to tell me I was experiencing anxiety but I said it felt much worse and there's no way it could be just anxiety. The doctor sat with me for a while and talked to me about anxiety and depression and felt it would be a good idea for me to go on antidepressants for a while. I initially refused because I didn't see the need. My then boyfriend and my Mum arrived at the hospital during this conversation with the doctor and he asked them if they had found my mood to be low.

They both agreed that I had been hard to get along with. This was news to me and I was alarmed. I telephoned my dad about the situation.

"I think everyone wants to put me in Belmont," I exclaimed. Belmont is a well-know psychiatric hospital in Brisbane. "I feel like everyone is ganging up on me."

In this situation Dad really came into his own. He just got it and drove down to Brisbane and took charge. Dad is really old-school and thinks a good night's rest will fix anything. But now he had a whole new understanding about MS and knew that what I was experiencing was anxiety over the life change that a chronic illness brings to you.

"You're not depressed mate," said Dad. "But we've got to get you through a few things first." He was amazing. Dad stayed at the hospital with me for a few days and gave me the strength I needed to try and get through that time. With Dad's calmness and sensibility to support me I thought 'what have I got to lose? Maybe I should just see how I feel by taking the antidepressants.'

I found that life was a lot tougher without the antidepressants. I was so embarrassed for a long time that I was taking medication for depression but then I realised the tablets help me get through the tough times that MS can bring. I can now manage shitty days better. And having a new baby can bring a lot of challenging days, let alone managing the MS symptoms on top of that.

Through Dad I learned that it was okay to have a good whinge and let off steam but then I had to pull my head in. For a while there I spent too much time feeling sorry for myself. And even now, I still have moments where I get really down. But I now know to put a time limit on those feelings. I literally wallow for an hour or two and then I say 'That's it. Get up. Have a shower and get over yourself.' If I didn't do that I think I'd end up in a downward spiral again. Sometimes if I've had a vent to my Dad about things I'll get a text message from him an hour or two later and it just says 'That's enough. You'll be alright.'

My Mum has also been my rock since the beginning and I'd be lost without her. She's always on the end of the phone for me and has found so many ways to help make my day-to-day life easier. I know in my heart she's breaking inside because of the diagnosis, but she's so brave. Now that I'm a mother myself I 'get it.' You would do anything to protect your children.

They say that tragedy brings people closer together and I certainly feel closer than ever to my parents and sisters. Their support has helped me form a new foundation for life and I have drawn my strength from them.

Perhaps because of the strong support from my family and friends I've become a really happy person now and I try not to let the little stuff bother me anymore. There will still be things that come up that I get cranky about but in the overall scheme I make sure I don't stay mad or depressed at things for too long. It's just a waste of time.

According to the National Multiple Sclerosis Society MS can affect more than just your physical abilities. It can also take a toll on your emotional health. Their research shows that half of all people living with multiple sclerosis struggle with clinical depression at some point during the course of their disease. It may be triggered by stress or grief, or it may actually be a result of brain atrophy caused by the MS itself.

It is also important to keep in mind that occasional feelings of sadness are normal for both people living with MS and their families. Depression is often hard to distinguish from grief. Persons with MS may experience losses—for example of the ability to work, to walk, or to engage in certain leisure activities. The process of mourning for these losses may resemble depression. However, grief is generally time-limited and resolves on its own. Moreover, a person experiencing grief may at times be able to enjoy some of life's activities. Clinical depression is more persistent and unremitting, with symptoms lasting at least two weeks and sometimes up to several months. It's important to distinguish between mild, everyday 'blues' that we all experience from time to time, grief, and clinical depression. Clinical depression, which must be diagnosed by a mental health professional, is a serious condition that produces flare-ups known as major depressive episodes.[3]

Signs of Depression in People Living With MS

People with multiple sclerosis who are feeling depressed might say they're feeling sad, glum, low, worthless, unwanted or like a failure. These are psychological signs of a depressive mood and are not unusual in people living with MS.

Sometimes symptoms of depression are physical. People might experience exhaustion, difficulty staying asleep, and changes in appetite.

People who are depressed often want to withdraw from activities and the resulting lack of stimulation further reduces their quality of life, creating a downward spiral. While supportive family and friends may help a person shake off mild depression, psychotherapy and/or antidepressant medication are generally needed to treat the condition adequately and prevent an even deeper depression that is harder to treat. Although support groups may offer some help with milder types of depression, they are not effective in treating severe clinical depression. Psychotherapy and/or antidepressant medication are more effective in treating severe clinical depression.

One of my coping mechanisms is to weigh up the consequences on the small stuff and only fight the battles that will actually gain something for everyone.

My diagnosis changed everything for me. It made me see things more clearly. The first thing I did was to get out of a relationship that wasn't working. My then boyfriend clearly wanted different things out of life and I wasn't willing to compromise or put things on hold any longer. It made me examine the sort of person I wanted to be with.

Husbands or partners fit into a different category to your parents or friends when it comes to dealing with your MS. Parents generally want to protect you and save you from everything a chronic illness brings. Friends are a great part of the support group, but they also have their own lives to go back to. A husband makes a very distinct choice to stay and support that woman for the rest of their lives together - possibly raising kids and making life choices that you don't make with your parents or friends.

We have this wall at home that we've painted with blackboard paint and divided into three separate lists. One is for the bottle and feed times, one is for the groceries and the last section is our list of dreams. We see it every day and it makes us remember why we're busting our butts and trying so hard to get our life together established. One of our goals is to build our own house. Barend is a builder and he's already designed our dream home to have the master suite on the ground floor. He's explained to me that if we did it that way, we'd have a great downstairs area that I could primarily live in and do all the day-to-day household things. He was looking ahead and planning for a workable area, just in case my mobility did become an issue. He wasn't shoving it in my face though; he actually sold it to me as a good floor plan to have in case our elderly parent came to stay with us! I think it may also have been a way he could take control of a situation that is hard to control.

If I ever talk to Barend about the MS and what the future may hold he always replies nonchalantly that he's fine with it. We never really talk about it in any detail. He agrees with me when I suggest we should see my psychologist together and talk about a few things but I know he never will. He's happy I see a psych, but he doesn't believe he needs to go himself. Men tend to just cope in silence. And to be honest, I'm now at the point where I can only be worried about me. My job is to be healthy and happy for our son Cooper, because without healthy parents, he suffers. With regards to the mental and emotional part of dealing with MS, I can only fix me, so that's all I can be worried about.

I truly believe that I've been given a child that is good and sweet and inherently knows I've got MS. On those days when I'm struggling I might say 'Oh Cooper, please be a good boy,' or 'Come and give Mummy a cuddle,' and he just knows. He'll give me the tightest hug or just go from tearing around the house to settling down a bit. I'm blessed to have a child who just seems to understand. He's only a toddler but he just seems to get it. What I've learned as a mum with MS is to pick the battles that I'm going to fight. And you know what, if it's a choice of having Cooper throwing a tantrum because I want to take a set of keys away, then really, what harm is it for him to play with the keys? What's to be gained from me taking a set of keys from him? That's just an example, but one of my coping mechanisms is to weigh up the consequences on the small stuff and only fight the battles that will actually gain something for everyone. Otherwise I don't sweat the small stuff. And that goes for everything, whether at home or work or socially. I pick my battles to conserve my energy for my family and the things that really matter to me.

I have learned to listen to my body. I used to push hard and then my body would crash the next day and I would realise I'd taken it too far. Now I know the signs and listen to them and I don't feel guilty about having a rest or asking for help. It's not always easy, but I know the consequences if I don't.

I'm really happy with the person I've become since my diagnosis of MS. I've had to learn to let go of the things that just aren't important. I've become more relaxed about a lot of things because of it. Living with MS makes you reconsider what really matters in life. I live more in the moment now. For me, it's all about what I choose to use my energy on wisely.

Regan's Tips for Living with MS

*"One of my coping mechanisms is to weigh up
the consequences on the small stuff and only fight
the battles that will actually gain something for everyone."*

- When you are first diagnosed you are so overwhelmed with what it all means for the future and you will likely turn to the internet for answers. Sometimes that can be a bad thing because it's Murphys Law for you to choose the site that shows someone in a wheelchair straight up!

- Don't be afraid to get a second opinion or seek out a different neurologist if you don't feel comfortable. You will see this person for a long time so you need to have a good relationship and feel like you are being heard.

- Make sure your family gets the information that your doctor or the MS Clinic will give you as it is extremely important that they understand what is happening.

- Seek out a good counsellor. Even if you don't feel you need one straight away, you will benefit from speaking to a professional at some point.

- Ask for help and accept it when it is offered!

- If and when you are ready to tell your employer, be honest with them; they will be more understanding of your situation when you need time off or need reduced duties.

- Keep up-to-date with research and clinical trials of MS cures. It will help keep you positive that the cure is getting closer!

- Get involved in fundraising. It's fun and you feel like you are helping yourself and others with this condition.

- Be as organised as you possibly can. Even small things such as having meals ready in advance on days you might work so everyone has a decent meal.

- My final tip would be to take the pressure off yourself and have a laugh! Surround yourself with positive, fun people who don't treat you any differently.

PAUL PISASALE

"You want to know the cure for MS? It's very simple. It's looking inside yourself. You hold the key to living a more successful and whole life. You can choose to lose control or you can choose to take control."

Born & bred in Ipswich, Paul Pisasale was elected to the city's Council in 1991, elected Deputy Mayor in 2000 and has served as the Mayor of the City of Ipswich for three successive terms since 2004. Lauded for his vision in transforming Ipswich into a bustling city in its own right, he demonstrated great leadership in managing his city through the 2011 floods – the worst flooding the State had ever seen. As a constant champion for his community, Paul was named Queensland's Local Hero for 2010 at the Australian of the Year Awards.

***

MS is no different to any other obstacle in life. You just need to make the decision on how to deal with it. We've got one life to live and you can either live every day of it happy or worrying. I always think to myself that the expectation of bad things happening is far worse than the actual event. I remember as a kid I was far more afraid waiting for the belting than actually receiving it! And MS is a lot like that. I used to sit around fearing when the next flare would occur. For the first year after my diagnosis I was constantly worrying about when it would attack again. But you know what?

Now that I've stopped worrying about it, the attacks have stopped happening.

Every time I have an MRI I live in hope that the brain lesions are disappearing. One has actually disappeared so I guess whatever I'm doing is working. I'm convinced it's my positive attitude and to be honest, I forget that I even have MS some days. I think your own mind can be the most dangerous thing when you've got MS. It would be easy to convince yourself that you're going to get sick.

In hindsight, I don't know how long I've had MS. But I can remember driving to the Gold Coast for a friend's party and on the way down, I felt the car drift to one side of the highway and I'd hit the side barrier. I wondered if I'd fallen asleep but it didn't really feel like that. When I arrived at the party I called my wife Janet and explained that I didn't think I should drive home that night.

"Come clean Paul," she joked. "If you want to stay down there and party with your mates just be honest."

"Janet, I'm not drunk at all, I'm just really tired. It's hard to explain," I said.

I drove back to Ipswich the next day and went straight to work. I was deputy mayor at the time. I was trying to sit through meetings but I just didn't feel right. My brother Charlie came in after the meeting to ask what was wrong.

"I'm just feeling very dizzy. It's probably nothing; just flu or something," I said. But then I got up to walk down the hallway to the next meeting and walked straight into a wall. I went back to my office to take a few aspirin and I put my head on the table. Next thing, I wake up and my brother had called for an ambulance and I was being taken to hospital.

One of my co-workers related to me much later that she remembers seeing me walk down the hallway and became alarmed. She said I was actually swaying, but it didn't look like I was drunk, it looked quite serious.

I was admitted to intensive care as the doctors were concerned

I might have been having a heart attack or stroke. After many cardiovascular tests one doctor suggested that they move onto neurological possibilities.

And by now everyone knows the ending to this story. The MRI displayed a collection of lesions on my brain and the neurologist declared I had MS. So I stayed in hospital for a few days.

Those first few days I felt life was over. "Why me?" I kept thinking. "This is not what I had planned for my life." When the neurologist broke the news to me that I had MS he urged me to look for a job that wasn't as stressful and didn't involve long hours. I wanted to become mayor and I felt I could kiss that one goodbye. I got my computer out and Googled 'MS.' That was the worst thing I could have done. I felt even more hopeless and just lay staring at the ceiling for hours. I guess I was in shock. Within such a short space of time everything had changed.

Later that day an elderly couple came into the ward to visit a friend. They saw me just lying there, staring despondently at the ceiling.

"What's wrong?" enquired the wife. I told them about the bad news I'd just been dealt. And as only someone of that generation could respond, she said "What are you worried about? You want to hear a bad story, I'll tell you a bad story." And she and her husband told me about all these other people who'd had bad things happen in life.

And she was right. There were people enduring far worse situations than me. It was enough to shake me out of my reverie. I called my staff and asked them to bring up some work. I wasn't about to lie there feeling sorry for myself any longer. I wanted to get back into things and figure it out as I went along.

During my time in hospital I actually had an important function I wanted to attend. It was the unveiling of a monument and I was meant to give a speech at the ceremony. The doctors wouldn't allow me to go. I ended up just getting dressed and walking out and after the ceremony I called my sister and asked her to meet me at the hospital. Luckily she walked in just as I was returning. The nurses were rushing around trying to find me and spotted us both.

"Where have you been Paul? We've been looking for you everywhere!" one nurse exclaimed.

With that I turned to my sister and asked, with a confused look on my face, "I'm really not sure.... Sis, where did you take me? Where did we go for our walk? I think I'd better go lie down now."

My sister was furious that I'd escaped and used her as an alibi.

***

About three years passed between my initial diagnosis and running for the Mayor of Ipswich. I was determined that the MS was not going to change me or stop me from what I wanted to do. The first time I ran for mayor in 2004 I got 60% of the vote and the second time in 2008 I got 88%. I was determined to get stronger and stronger and I did.

Do you remember that popular television show starring Martin Sheen called The West Wing? I had become Mayor at the same time that programme was showing the episode about how the President of the United States was coming out to the public with his MS.

I remember the plot went along the lines of exploring whether President Jed Bartlett had deceived the people of America. Until that point I hadn't really considered if my diagnosis was impacting the people of Ipswich or not. All of a sudden I was thinking twice about it and worried whether I should have disclosed my medical condition. After a lot of self-reflection I figured the difference between the American president and myself was that I didn't have my finger on the nuke button!

Coincidentally, a well-known journalist named Madonna King called me at this time. Madonna is described as the 'voice of current affairs in Brisbane,' and I respected her. She said that she had heard through friends that I'd been helping other people with MS and she asked point blank if I was living with MS and would I come onto her radio program and speak about it? I was very quiet while I contemplated what she said.

"No, I don't think I'm ready for that," I answered.

"But I really think you could help a lot of people if you told your story," she explained.

I went away and thought about the request for 48 hours. To be honest, I was still a bit embarrassed about having MS. I was worried about what people would think about it and I also worried about people drawing the wrong conclusions as to my abilities. The problem with MS is that there's a lot of misconception out there as to what it is and how it affects people.

But I called her back and agreed to do the interview and the rest is history. Since coming out, people from everywhere approach me about the topic. I met a young photographer not long after that Madonna King interview. He came up to me at an exhibition I was attending, sat next to me and told me that we shared the same neurologist. He'd been diagnosed the previous year and he told me that the thing that helped him was knowing that I had it. It was tremendously humbling to hear that.

I really don't know what the public perception was to my 'coming out'. I don't know whether people felt deceived; but not long after my announcement I got 82% of the vote in the mayoral election so my guess is that my electorate felt pretty comfortable with me doing the job.

When I first thought about coming out publicly with the fact I had MS I was concerned people would think it was a publicity stunt. I was afraid they'd think I was after a sympathy vote. Ten years ago, people were still being fired from their jobs because of disabilities. The stigma was very strong that people living with MS weren't able to function properly. I went on the warpath with that misconception. I won't stand for it and I want it eradicated. I've met some employers who are scared to shake hands with people with MS because they think it's contagious.

Having MS has made me a better person, although I don't advocate getting MS to become a better person! But you've got to understand that in life everyone has their own issues to deal with. And if we don't support each other enough in how we deal with the issues then we're doomed as a society. I've learned a new sense of compassion and that's why I simply don't tolerate employers who won't work with people affected by MS. Employment is about dignity and achieving a goal in life. I'm living proof that a person with MS can not only do the job, but in fact do a better job. I think we become more determined to show everyone that we can achieve excellent results.

Not long ago I got thirty people together who had MS and we made sure they had a forum to talk about the positive things they'd done. It gave everyone inspiration to go out and do even better things with their life. I had one woman come up to me after the event and exclaim that she wished she had MS! She was that moved by how many people had turned their life around.

The first MS support group I ever went to was a different story; it made me feel really depressed afterwards. It was a lot of people sitting around complaining and I just know there are people worse off than us out there. My own support group is my immediate family and a close group of friends who not only check in on me, but also keep me grounded and make sure I'm striving for that work/life balance. I really don't need to talk about my MS and its condition at all, but it's nice knowing I have people keeping their eye out for me.

Prior to my diagnosis I felt I was bullet-proof. Probably a lot of men do. Men are idiots when it comes to speaking about their emotions or communicating with their wife or their staff. I'm trying to be a better communicator, but my own team know me really well and know I'm a dramatic and emotional Italian. But since the diagnosis I think I've become more sensitive and understanding as a person and I also think I achieve more now because I trust my team to support me in getting things done. I've definitely become a better delegator. Given that I have to guard my time and energy due to the sheer workload that comes with being mayor but also because of the MS, I've had to learn delegation and time management skills as a survival tactic.

Taking up golf has become a great outlet for me and also good physical therapy. Everyone thinks I'm playing against them when I play in a match, but I'm not – I'm paying against myself. In a way, I concentrate harder when playing golf because I want to win or improve my score and prove that people with MS can still be champions. I also like winning and letting people know that someone with MS beat them!

I once did a MS Moonlight Walk with Robert de Castella, the World and Commonwealth Games Champion marathon runner. As we were nearing the finish line I turned to Robert and said "It's been really great doing this event with you Robert and I hope what I'm about to do doesn't cause a rift in our friendship."

"What do you mean Paul? What's going on?" asked Robert.

"Well, it's just that sometimes I do things that are more driven by ego than common sense."

And with that I took off, raised my arms in a victory pose and raced across the finish line yelling "I just beat Robert de Castella! How's it feel to get beaten by someone with MS buddy?" He just shook his head and laughed and laughed.

MS is a different type of disease. It can be really hard to talk about living with MS. When you have something that changes how you go about things you don't necessarily want to talk about it to your friends because you don't want them to think of you any differently. You don't want them to think you're less capable or feel sorry for you. But on the flip side, you need some understanding and occasionally some assistance. And particularly as a man you don't want to burden your family and friends. You just want to get on with things.

Having MS had made me change quite a bit about how I live life now. I decided not to deliver prepared speeches as I found it too nerve wracking to try and memorise everything, but rather I speak from the heart. I spend some time understanding the group or situation I'm presenting to and talk to them with spontaneity.

If I have ceremonies where I know there's going to be a lot of names to read out I'll get my fellow councillors to assist. The Australia Day citizenship ceremonies are a good example. I'm so honoured to be presiding over these occasions but I'll get a councillor to read the names of our new citizens and I'll assist in presenting their citizenship certificates. My fellow councillors love to be involved so it's a win-win situation. They think it's great that I share the ceremonial duties around.

If I have functions that require following a very strict protocol, I'd rather not do it or my staff will develop a work-around. I'm mainly concerned with offending people if I have a memory lapse in what's meant to happen and frankly, I don't need the additional stress. But who does? My staff are amazing people. They've become tremendously adaptive in working with me. I probably don't know half of what they engineer in the background. But they look out for me without making a big deal about it. MS has taught me to trust a bit more. I have learned to let go of things that I don't need to control and let others take the reins. I think the culture of the council has changed tremendously because of it.

In my role, I get a lot of invitations to attend functions, particularly at night. It's an important part of being the mayor - to be the public face of our great city. But I can't physically go to all of them and I do have to be sensibly protective of my energy. So now I film video messages that can be played at the events. I was worried that the guests might think it was a bit of a cop out, but they love it. The hosts can play the message whenever it fits into their program and they've got an enduring piece of media that they can use on their websites. I can still put the same compassion and heart into my messages. In a way, the council is now better represented in the community because we've thought outside the square in how to get things done. While guarding my energy because of the MS may have been the premise for devising solutions, the advantages for the community and workplace as a whole have been tremendous. They're probably changes that should have happened regardless of me having MS, but it was the diagnosis that forced me to think about doing things differently.

Living with MS is all about finding adaptive techniques. And you can actually make your life better. I hear stories all the time about people who have made such positive changes in their life or change their career completely because of the MS. These are happy people.

Paul's Tips for Living with MS

"I think your own mind can be the most dangerous thing when you've got MS. It would be easy to convince yourself that you're going to get sick."

You want to know the cure for MS? It's very simple. It's looking inside yourself. You hold the key to living a more successful and whole life.

It's how you tackle the disease head on and how you choose to view how the symptoms affect you. You can choose to lose control or you can choose to take control.

Life deals out cards to people that sometimes seem unfair. And the trouble we get ourselves into is when we expect a certain card to be dealt and it doesn't happen. And when something different happens it can throw your whole life out of control. And that happened to me....

But I only let it happen to me for a day. I was lucky that I had enough people around me to convince me that nothing needed to change. My legs are still working; my arms are stilling working; and my brain is still working; so I have to be grateful for that.

As Australians we treat things differently. We're all larrikins and our way of dealing with some of the tough things in life is to laugh at ourselves and make fun of it. I don't want the MS to define me in any way, otherwise it means I'm playing by someone else's rules. It's human nature to feel sorry for yourself occasionally, but what I've learned is not to wallow too long. Give it a few minutes and move on.

So the thing now is to just get on with life. We don't know how life works and what's going to happen tomorrow, but if you treat each day with misery then you're just wasting a valuable day that someone else gave you.

LINDA EDGERTON

"Taking actions to improve my overall health and seeing the results on my MS was empowering."

....

Sometimes you can be cruising along living a seemingly 'normal' happy life, but it's only in hindsight you see the struggle. For me, being diagnosed with Multiple Sclerosis in 2002 brought more relief than shock. Finally there was an explanation for the not-quite-right health I'd been pushing through for years. I instantly became gentler on myself. Now I could fully appreciate what I had achieved and be more focussed and patient about every aspect of my future life. I would learn to manage my symptoms and energy, and make choices that reflected my values and passions. MS would be a catalyst to improving my life.

Like many people with MS, the road to diagnosis was a confusing maze. Looking back, my first MS symptoms began much earlier. In the years leading to diagnosis I often experienced overwhelming fatigue; physical and mental exhaustion that appeared suddenly for no reason. This was very different to tiredness brought on by effort or lack of sleep. I'd also struggle on hot days, always seeking out the shade. Sometimes white spots appeared before my eyes then they'd disappear. Weird sensations throughout my body also came and went. Then in May 2002, I experienced tingling in my lips and chin area. Since I was about to travel to Africa, I enquired to the doctor about this and was told it was probably stress. I remember thinking, "that's strange, it's not a stressful time." Five months – and many symptoms and tests later – I would be diagnosed with MS.

My response to being diagnosed with MS was greatly influenced by previous personal challenges. Severe glandular fever at age 20 saw me return home from university and bed-ridden for months. A very driven person, I had tried to push on and then crashed further, my confidence plummeting in the same direction as my health. I was given no treatment and received little understanding outside my immediate family. The doctor had unhelpfully told me "it's just glandular fever, you won't die." I didn't know how to get help. I spent the next few years struggling through my study, work and social life, a changed person who felt very disconnected. It was a complex act of balancing energy and output during this time. I dreamt a lot about experiencing life and seeing the world. My dad's sudden death from a heart attack (at age 54 when I was 27) reminded me how short and precious life is. By the time I was diagnosed with multiple sclerosis at age 37, I had amassed many incredible memories as well as a satisfying career. With the MS diagnosis, I didn't have that fear of being left behind or missing out that I'd felt when I had glandular fever at the age of 20. This time I would also access the support team I needed. I felt confident that life could recover. With patience, adjustment, learning, effort and new dreams, I would maintain inner peace and a joy for life.

Perspective also changes things. Five days after my MS diagnosis, the Bali bombings killed 202 people, including 88 Australians, many of them so very young. My future hadn't been taken from me. Surrounded by loved ones and with the best of medical care, life still offered me so much possibility – and responsibility.

The MS diagnosis and life journey is a very individual thing; we each experience MS differently and have our own ways of coping. My road to diagnosis began during a safari to Kenya and Tanzania in June 2002. The tingling in my lips and jaw that I'd experienced just before the trip became more constant and I started to have stabbing pain down the left side of my face. Later this symptom would have a label – trigeminal neuralgia. It's the most disturbing symptom I've experienced and 10 years later I still get it sometimes because treatment came so late. The numbness and less-severe pings I now experience have actually become one of my measures of wellness; they appear as an accurate warning sign of whenever I am run down and need extra self-care and rest. I treat these times as a 'health crisis' and do everything I can to calm my body and mind. Ironically, having this residual symptom (and others) has probably helped me to prevent further relapses.

While the facial symptoms I experienced in Africa were worrying, it was the addition of strong pain in my left leg and left arm that made me see a doctor. It felt like an aching bone in my lower leg and my arm had a burning sensation. In typical MS style, at first it came and went. I was trying hard to ignore the symptoms as I wanted to enjoy my trip. My immediate fear was that I'd picked up a tropical disease (immunisations don't cover all the possibilities). With the symptoms getting stronger with each day, I became increasingly anxious. When we reached the western highlands of Kenya, we were staying in a campsite located in the midst of a tea plantation in Kericho. The town was nearby and late in the evening I knew I had to find a doctor. Around midnight a taxi picked me up and took me to a very modern-looking hospital. Many people were out in the streets, so it felt surreal to walk into a hospital that was deserted except for a few staff. The doctor and nurse who saw me treated me with great kindness. I remember being apologetic for being there, I didn't want to be an over-dramatic westerner in a place where so many people needed care (we'd been passing signs with monthly malaria death statistics that had shocked me). The doctor was highly accomplished and had just returned from a conference in Spain where he'd been a speaker on AIDS. He tested me for stoke and asked many questions. We rang my insurance company and an Australian doctor then rang back. Together the doctors discussed my case. I was told it wasn't life threatening and was probably a pinched nerve, but I should see a doctor for more tests when I got home. They put my mind at ease. I only had a few days left on the trip so was happy to be given painkillers and to continue on (the logistics of trying to leave early were too overwhelming considering it wasn't necessary). The capsules were effective in easing my pain and the insurance company was delighted to add this doctor as a new contact for the Kericho area. My strongest memory is of the nurse and me waiting in the room for the doctor, our arms held out next to each other admiring the two colours together. "You're beautiful," "No, you're beautiful," "We're beautiful!"

On the plane home I focused more on the symptoms I was feeling, which now included a constant headache. I felt massive relief to be home and that night went to the hospital emergency room. The doctor just confirmed it wasn't life threatening and told me to make an appointment with my GP. That appointment led to a month's wait to see a neurologist. To be able to continue on with work, I took the maximum allowed dose of neurofen during this time, something I wouldn't recommend as it can cause stomach problems. Many possible causes were slowly eliminated. Finally, in early October (after being very patient with the medical system), I was at the reception desk after an appointment with the neurologist and broke down in tears saying, "I'm not going home, I don't feel safe". I felt so much pain, was frightened I was dying and just couldn't cope anymore. I needed answers – and help. They put me in hospital that day. I had MRIs on my brain and spine, a lumbar puncture and other tests, and was finally given the diagnosis of MS. I was given the three-day infusion treatment of methylprednisolone (anti-inflammatory steroids), which had immediate results. The pain eased (but never completely as some scarring must have remained). When I had the steroids the following year for numbness along my right side, I had complete recovery. Swift treatment definitely makes a difference.

The level of stress I felt during the months leading to diagnosis was insane. I'd returned straight to full-time work after my holiday. Despite having more than four months of unused sick leave accrued (I'd worked in communications roles in universities for years and had carried this leave over several positions), my workload was intense and I felt very uncomfortable taking days off for appointments. I was bringing work home just to keep up. After my eight-day hospital stay, which involved two weeks off work, I felt I had to tell my manager and colleagues about my diagnosis. They were all very caring and concerned. I was keen to put on a brave face, stop the attention and get some normality back in my life. Looking back, it was ridiculous I wasn't given more time off work. When you have sick leave accrued, shouldn't it be available for physical healing and emotional adjustment after being diagnosed with a serious incurable disease? Without the doctors giving me more sick leave (or me having the clarity of mind to ask for it), the only way to manage stress and slowly rebuild my health and endurance was to make my life outside work very 'small' for a couple of years – work, meals, rest, sleep. I continued to have a range of odd sensory symptoms that would come and go, the weirdest were chest tightness (known as the 'MS hug') and Lhermitte's sign (electric shocks travelling down the spine, this one was so bizarre it kind of fascinated me). These new symptoms were on and off for just a few days and I didn't have treatment or time off. Like my other symptoms, they were invisible to others. I was functioning and received excellent work reviews so it appeared I was back to 'normal'.

In late 2003, I was fortunate to hear about and attend a Gawler Foundation MS retreat led by Ian Gawler and Professor George Jelinek, author of Overcoming MS. This retreat included research-based advice about medication, nutrition, exercise, meditation and managing stress. It gave me the knowledge to assist in my own healing. As well as improving my physical health, learning to live in the present and to let go of fear, anger and sadness was a great help emotionally. Taking actions to improve my overall health and seeing the results on my MS was empowering. It took away that feeling of being out of control. Being committed to cooking and eating healthy meals, daily walks, getting some sunshine, meditation, nurturing connections – these things also created more joy in my life.

In 2004, two years after diagnosis, I was able to take three months long service leave. This time of rest, tranquillity and fun was incredibly healing; my health stabilised and has stayed that way ever since. I haven't had an MS relapse for over eight years and no longer take medication. Ten years after diagnosis, I still work full-time.

I have mixed feelings about disclosing MS in the workplace. After I shared I had MS I was given a 'case manager' in Human Resources. At a meeting with the case manager and my manager, they tried to get me to change to part-time work. I pointed out that I was already back working full-time, was capable of working full-time and needed to work full-time. I was then given a form for my doctor to fill out, which I gave back to them. My medical details were none of their business since the neurologist and GP had decided I was able to work full-time (if that turned out not to be the case, I had months of sick leave I could use at full pay). I may have imagined it, but I felt I had to perform above and beyond in my work to prove I was not affected by MS.

In my next two positions, I did not disclose MS as I knew I was more than capable of doing the work and didn't want any possible negative stigma and added pressure. It saddens me to caution the newly-diagnosed in this way as it's only through seeing people with MS perform well in the workforce that MS can be better understood and the path made easier for others. Unless you need adjustments made, perhaps just reveal MS when you've already proven yourself in your work. It's a personal decision. One of the hardest things with revealing MS is the people who look at you like something dire is going to happen. You certainly don't need that in a new workplace if you can avoid it. In my personal life, I've always shared that I have MS and have tried hard to increase people's understanding of the condition.

In the year after diagnosis I would wake every morning and the first thing that popped into my head would be "I have MS." It was my daily reality check that things were different, my future uncertain. The same thought would arise throughout the day.

Gradually over time I became more accepting and hopeful and now it's rare for me to ponder the fact I have MS. I don't fear it. Of course, it helps that my MS has been stable for a long period of time, but I never take that for granted. Life is more than MS and life is unpredictable for everyone.

Experience has taught me that wonderful things can happen at any age, including after times of deep sadness or turmoil. It might take longer to reach your dreams due to the interruptions of MS, but you're probably going to be so much clearer in what you seek and you'll appreciate it more when you get there. Relish the journey and don't underestimate the joys of small everyday pleasures – the life you can enjoy right now. The older I get the more I see simplicity as the secret to happiness. Work out what makes your heart full.

Linda's tips for healthy living after being diagnosed with MS

"Sleep is wonderful for healing."

Above everything else, make sure you get the sleep and rest you need, especially during a relapse or when you're run down from the demands of your work and life. Sleep is wonderful for healing. Try not to be frustrated that this means missing out on some things, you can make up for it when your health improves. Avoid rash decisions based on how you feel during a relapse. Welcome any support from family and friends, and hang in there with work and other commitments, even if this means going to bed at 8pm (I did that for the first year while I slowly improved my health).

***

Know that having MS does not make you 'less' in any way - the learning and inner-strength that comes from it can help you redirect and enjoy your life even more. Be resilient. Make adjustments to your life if needed, and at the same time ask yourself what you hope for next. Design new dreams so that you always have something to aim towards and look forward to. Continue to drink deep from the cup of life. Experiencing life's lows make the happy times all the more precious.

***

Keep your neurologist and GP fully informed about any complementary therapies you wish to try. Listen to their advice, then make your own choices.

***

Make healthy lifestyle choices. Nourish your body with whole foods, drink water, get out into the fresh air and enjoy some sunshine.

***

Use to-do lists. When your mind is racing, keep a diary – it helps get the thoughts out of your head. Meditation is calming, healing and easy to do (even 10 minutes a day helps).

***

Minimise contact with people who deplete rather than nourish you. Try to stay away from people with infections. Let family and friends know you need to protect your health as best you can and you'd appreciate if they could reschedule catch-ups if they have a cold/flu/bug. On public transport move seats if you notice person next to you is unwell. If you're getting recurring colds, rest properly and have lots of juices and green smoothies. Staying well with MS is supported by staying well in your general health.

***

Register with the MS Society to be kept updated about information sessions, support groups and research. Consider using the peer support service (I joined a group when first diagnosed and later became a one-to-one phone peer support volunteer for several years)

***

Plan travel carefully to include rest. Always take out travel insurance for overseas travel, with MS covered (it will cost more, but worth the peace of mind).

DIANNE HART

"I have MS but MS does not have me."

....

I was sworn into the Queensland Police Service in 1973 and then became a non-operational sergeant in 1990. I really love my job and over the years have had the opportunity to work in a number of administrative and frontline support roles such as Property and Exhibits, Crime Shoppers and my current position supporting the Cold Case Investigation Unit within the Homicide Squad.

Three decades ago the police force was fairly male dominated and not the easiest work environment for a female. There was still a lot of sexism and everything that goes along with it and I had probably been feeling stressed a bit from work. I woke up on Australia Day in 1986, rostered to work at a police function, but I had lost all vision in my right eye.

When my sight didn't return after a day or two I finally went and saw a GP who ran all the regular blood tests but didn't really come up with anything. He referred me onto an ophthalmologist who then referred onto a neurologist, who similarly didn't say much but advised me to go back to work for now because I'd need a lot of time off later. Curiously he also suggested that I should consider being very discreet about how I was feeling. He confirmed that it wasn't a brain tumour or anything like that, but I was a bit confused as to what was wrong. He never actually mentioned MS but I later found out he'd sent a letter to my ophthalmologist stating that he had diagnosed me as having multiple sclerosis.

I went on scheduled holidays after seeing the neurologist and tried to put everything out of my mind as best as possible, but when I experienced some further symptoms a few months later I went back to my GP who simply put everything down to having a virus. I was experiencing fatigue like I'd never felt before and had also lost sensation in my legs. It was actually a colleague at work who urged me to go and get a second opinion because he thought that what I was feeling was far more serious than the flu.

So I saw a new GP who reviewed all the other blood tests my previous doctor had ordered and agreed with me that what I had wasn't Ross River Fever or one of the other viral infections that were rampant in Australia at that time. He referred me to yet another neurologist. I was insistent on seeing an alternate neurologist as I was still very confused as to why the previous one had sent me away without an explanation.

The new neurologist performed a Visually Evoked Response test. The Visually Evoked Response test (VER), also known as the Visually Evoked Potential test (VEP), is a test for Optic Neuritis and other demyelinating events along the Optic Nerve or further back along the optic pathways.

The test involves watching a black and white checkered pattern on a TV screen in a darkened room. The black and white squares alternate on a regular cycle, which generates electrical potentials along the optic nerve and into the brain. These can be detected with electroencephalographical (EEG) sensors placed at specific sites on the top of the head (the occipital scalp). Each eye is tested independently while an eye patch is worn on the other eye.

VEPs are very sensitive at measuring slowed responses to visual events and can often detect dysfunction that is undetectable through clinical evaluation or if the person is unaware of any visual defects. Because of their ability to detect silent lesions and historic demyelinating episodes, they are very useful diagnostic tools.

Both the GP and neurologist suspected I could have either

Guillain-Barre Syndrome or Multiple Sclerosis. Guillain-Barre Syndrome (GBS) is an autoimmune disease where the body's immune system begins to attack the peripheral nervous system. I could see how my symptoms might have led them to conclude I had either of the conditions.

"Well the news is good Dianne," said the neurologist after examining all my results. "You don't have Guillain-Barre Syndrome but you do have Multiple Sclerosis. What do you know about MS?"

"Basically nothing," I replied. I remember being in a bit of shock. "But I do know you don't die from it."

He wrote me up a prescription for prednisone and told me to take it if I thought I was having another attack.

While all this was going on another colleague at work also suspected I had MS. Thirty years ago there was so little known about the condition but this colleague approached me one day and brought up the possibility.

"Don't you watch Neighbours?" asked the friend. 'Neighbours' is a popular television soap opera that started airing in Australia and the UK from 1985 and still runs today. "I reckon you've got exactly what Helen's sister has." To be honest, that was the first time I'd ever hear the words 'MS.' I started watching Neighbours from then on!

So after the neurologist told me what I had I went to the library, but all the books in the library were ancient and there was nothing to assist. I was so in the dark about what I had and what MS meant that when I visited a friend's place shortly after my diagnosis I refused to touch her kids. I'd always considered these children to be family but now I was dead-afraid of passing anything on. I just had no idea; I was in a cloud.

Thirty years ago no one really knew what to do. I don't think the doctors really wanted to deal with chronic illness or coaching people how to get on with life or where to find information. They didn't understand much about a condition like MS and back then had zero training in how to answer the hard questions from patients. On top of this, there weren't actually a lot of treatment options anyway. Prednisone - or steroids - were all that was on offer and that was only to soften the symptoms of an attack, not to prevent progression.

At the time of my diagnosis I never made a formal announcement to work about what I had. I think they probably knew though. Whenever I had any time off work my GP simply wrote it up as a 'viral infection.' It was a different time back then and I feared that if I had disclosed to my superiors that I had MS they would have ordered me out of the service as medically unfit. It wasn't until the early nineties that I did finally mention it to my direct manager but I urged her not to say anything to anyone. I didn't want special treatment. I just wanted to get on with my job.

Luckily it's a far different story now and those people who want and are able to continue working generally don't run up against too many issues. No one wants to think that they'd have to resort to legal action but there is legislation in place these days to ensure we get a fair deal at work.

It can be hard to decide if and when to tell people at work and only you will know the answer. But it's possible that by not saying anything your managers and co-workers may be thinking something even worse. They may think you're lazy or ambivalent. I'd rather have the correct label put on me, even if it is MS, than an inaccurate one. I'd rather be in control of what information people had than the alternative.

Now that I have been up front with my MS it's actually a bit easier. But I did have to wait for the right time and place to make my diagnosis public knowledge. I often carry a few of the booklets about MS around with me so that if people do have questions or are concerned about what I can and can't do – especially in the workplace – then they can read a booklet and get a general idea. It was a good starting point to educate people and I was always happy to answer further questions. Over the years there have been a few other people in the Force diagnosed and I seem to be their first stop in talking about how to get on with life once you've got MS.

I don't think the stigma attached to MS has changed that much over the years because I don't think we know much more about the disease itself. It's still a mystery disease to most people. It's quite funny that everybody knows someone with MS but no one really knows anything about the condition itself.

Fatigue has been my worst symptom and that's what I'm most diligent about managing. I have relapsing remitting MS (RRMS) but that doesn't mean I'm absolutely on top of things in the times when I'm not having a flare. You can feel quite severe symptoms without it being declared a flare or exacerbation. If it's particularly hot or I've pushed myself too hard my fatigue or eyesight might get worse. So every day you need to guard against letting the symptoms get worse.

Generally I just travel along as normal until I hit a wall. And to be honest, I often think I must have a pretty good version of RRMS. But once I hit that wall, I know I have to make resting and recovering a priority, so as I can get back up on my feet more quickly. My workplace has been exceptional at accommodating me when I need a bit of time off but I've never given less than 110% when I'm at work so my managers know that everything is going to get done.

But the flip side of my commitment to work is that I limit my socialising. Some of my social life over the years has been dampened due to the shift work I've had to do but I also recognise that I can't do it all. While I'm living with MS I can't give 100% of myself to work and also 100% to a social life. But who can?

Everyone's symptoms of MS and how they live with it are different, so it's important to set your own priorities in how you deal with things. My own garden at home is a bit of a mess because I decided that having a picture-perfect garden was not the most important thing to me. Instead I wanted to concentrate on getting my rest so I could work. It gives me far more satisfaction.

I've been very fortunate to have a best friend who's been with me through the thick and thin of MS. She's been there when I needed to have a good cry or to vent and also celebrate the triumphs too. I can't stress enough how important it is to find your support group when you have MS. Whether it's a friend, a family member or a formal group that you attend you will need a person you can talk to or trust to be there when you need it.

I'm a fairly self-assured person but some days the MS eats away at my confidence a bit. When you're an independent woman used to doing everything you want and then you find yourself having to judge on a daily basis if doing something now will be at the detriment to having energy later it can knock your confidence around a bit. It's a constant juggling act of second-guessing yourself.

This feeling can really depend on where you are in life. The times when I've been in a really great role and a happy work environment, it's been easier to feel like I can take on the world. But in those times when additional stress was placed on me I found my confidence eroded and I'd get tired and cranky much more easily. Now that might be the situation for anyone in a stressful situation, but when you have MS loaded on top of your regular stressors it's hard not to run yourself ragged. You're trying to do your job in a tense situation, keep the peace, do the normal things in life that everyone has to do, like pay the bills, eat and sleep AND on top of that you need to protect your health against the MS. It's too many things wanting to take a piece out of you and something's got to give. If you want to work successfully with MS it's vital that you don't do it in a place with undue stress. You just won't excel and you'll sabotage your health.

I think the biggest and most positive impact you can make on your health is to eliminate all the stress. Having the will to say 'no' when you're feeling unwell could mean that you take one day off from your regular activities rather than three. It's all about being kind to yourself. There will be days when you absolutely can't control what's happening to you body but those are the days when you need to just sit back and go with the flow.

The body is tremendously good at repairing itself if you give it the proper tools. Something as simple as a good night of sleep can do wonders.

I decided years ago not to continue with any medication. I've tried a few different ones and I just felt worse whilst taking them. My neurologist felt very strongly that I was making a bad decision to come off treatment but I'm firm in believing that I make all the final decisions about my body. Just because I'm not on medication doesn't mean I don't think they work. For me it was a choice of weighing up what the side effects might do to me compared to the benefit of taking the medication. I felt like I was already dealing with enough in my life without dealing with additional issues. But it's different for everyone. It's a very personal decision to make and I wouldn't take it lightly. Do your research and weigh up the pros and cons of the various medications and their side effects. There are so many options out there now compared to 30 years ago.

I strongly believe in the power of positive thinking. You might have MS but it doesn't have you. If you become too wrapped up in everything that's wrong and only talk to other people who have MS then you'll go down very quickly. I've seen it time-after-time in my nearly three decades of living with MS. You have to be vigilant with your energy but you can't live and breathe MS.

I personally feel that it's your own mental attitude towards the MS that will determine how well you cope with it. It's as simple as that. The people who fight it have a much better quality of life; they live longer and they get more out of life.

I look at MS like climbing Mt Everest. Sometimes I might stumble, but that's fine, I'll keep going. Sometimes I might even fall, but I'll sit for a moment and brush myself off until I'm ready to get up and go again. And sometimes I fall right to the very bottom. But with a bit of reflection and rest I get the energy and courage to get up and start climbing again.

Dianne's Tips to Living with MS

- When you receive the dreaded news that you have MS you will experience many different emotions from fear to questioning your future and wondering if you'll end up in a wheelchair. Try not to give these emotions any more time than needed. It's counter-productive.

- Be thankful that you only have MS and not some other medical condition that could, in fact, take your life.

- Once you have recovered from your first experience of MS be positive about your continued recovery because no one knows how it will affect you. You may never have another episode or you may experience a number of exacerbations, one after the other. It affects each of us differently.

- There are a number of symptoms and you may experience only one or a number of them. And this may continue to change over time. Take control of your body and get to know what may trigger an exacerbation. Keep a journal of your symptoms.

- Lack of sleep will cause fatigue. Doing too much physical activity could also drain your energy.

- Learn to take a break or ask for assistance.

- Learn to say no because taking a few hours now is better than needing a few days to recover later.

- Don't over-consume alcohol because this will only make your symptoms worse and it may cause depression.

- If you are experiencing fatigue due to the heat consider using cooling devices such as a gel wrap around your neck or a cooling vest.

- Don't get over heated in the winter by rugging up or cranking the heating too high. Even taking very hot showers in winter may cause your symptoms to flare up.

- Hydro-therapy and water sports can be a great alternative to going to the gym because the water supports your body and allows you to remain cooler so you can exercise for longer.
- I've found that regular meditation and Reike have been great tools in controlling my symptoms.
- Don't be afraid to have a good cry as a way of letting things go. For me it's a bit like a cleansing.
- If you get involved in an organised support group, make sure it has a really positive vibe. Negativity breeds a negative attitude, which will affect your health. Supportive groups help to provide information on the different symptoms that you may be experiencing and provide suggestions on how to manage them.

NICOLE JUBBER

"Letting go of that feeling of having to get everything done feels a bit like losing control, but really it's all about gaining control; gaining control of your own time, health and wellbeing."

I've always been an incredibly motivated person; someone who was always running around getting things done. But I did feel like I was always on the hamster wheel. Peddling; peddling; peddling.... but there was always still more 'stuff' to get through. Given this analogy of my life, it was probably no wonder I was given the run-around in getting my diagnosis of MS.

I know that from the age of 25 onwards I experienced a lot of different viral infections, be it ear, chest or sinus. They would just come and go. Despite this, I wasn't an unhealthy person, I think I was just always getting these infections because I was too busy to properly look after myself. Around this time I was working as a human resources manager for the National Australia Bank in Melbourne. I'm not sure what brought it on and exactly how to describe the symptoms, but I had a severe attack of dizziness and was taken to the Alfred Hospital where I stayed for five days. The doctors performed test after test to try and figure out what was wrong. They explained that if I did all these tests as an outpatient, it would take months, so it was best to be admitted and have everything performed at once.

I had various scans and a lumbar puncture, did balance exercises and sensory testing. After a few days both the lumbar puncture and

MRI tests came back with results that indicated MS. However my doctors were reluctant to actually call the diagnosis definitively at that point and to this day I still don't understand why. Perhaps it was because this was the first time I'd presented to hospital with the symptoms and they wanted to wait for a second attack.

So in the end they sent me home with the alternative diagnosis of migraines and advised me to come back to hospital for another MRI if it ever happened again. It was awful! After days of tests and going through a pretty horrific experience I was still none the wiser as to why I was experiencing these symptoms. Looking back, why wouldn't they have even mentioned the possibility of MS to me rather than just making it a notation on my chart? It must have been in their mind for them to urge me to come back for an MRI.

Over the next five years I suffered through a lot of migraines and dizzy spells and also experienced a deep fatigue. I saw a kinesiologist and an acupuncturist; I went on special diets and cut out dairy and gluten... I basically put myself through 101 different tests and did so many extreme things trying to fix myself along with various practitioners to try to work out why I felt so tired and kept getting severe headaches.

And while nothing was extremely debilitating, a few times a year my husband wouldn't be able to go to work because he felt he needed to stay at home and keep an eye on me. But life more or less carried on regardless. I kept wondering why I was so tired and experiencing the dizzy spells and headaches but after a while I just put it down to the stress of life. By this stage I had two young daughters and really felt that I just had to get on with things no matter what. Then one night in 2006, about five years after the first episode, I was refereeing a netball game and the world started spinning. I could feel an extremely severe dizzy attack coming on and was basically taken off the field. But this felt different to the other attack I'd experienced previously and additional symptoms also started manifesting. Over the next 72 hours I started losing sensation in different parts of my body. I was walking with a loopy gait and the fatigue was extreme.

After three days of this I finally went to my GP who then referred me to a neurologist in Geelong for an MRI. When the results were in, I clearly remember this neurologist striding in to the exam room and announcing with absolutely no compassion or bedside manner that I had benign MS. I was in shock. What was benign MS? What did it mean and what did I need to do? Before I could ask any more questions, he explained to me dismissively that I could go now but to certainly come back if anything happened again!

In the following days I recounted this story to my family. My sister couldn't believe what had happened and told me it wasn't good enough. She urged me to find another specialist in Melbourne and to get better answers and direction.

Benign MS is a label that was developed for people who live with MS for years without developing any disabilities at all.

Like so much else in MS, no one understands why some MS is so mild. Even the proportion of people with benign MS is unclear. Estimates range from 5 to 40 percent in different studies and some doctors have even called for a halt in the use of this term.

However everyone agrees that benign describes the very mildest form of MS. These people have had enough neurological symptoms and MRI abnormalities to be diagnosed — but for the next ten to twenty years their physical disability is mild to nonexistent.

Whether a neurologist agrees or disagrees about the use of the term 'benign MS' Dr John R. Richert, MD, an American neurologist and head of the National Multiple Sclerosis Society's research and clinical programs explains good reason to take action. "Right now, the best advice we can give is to get on an MS therapy as soon as possible following a definite diagnosis of MS with active disease, and for many, even after experiencing a first attack that puts them at high risk for developing MS," said Dr. Richert. "At the time of diagnosis and for years thereafter, it is impossible to know if the disease will be benign or more active and early treatment is the best defence we have for slowing this disease." [4]

I took my sister's advice to get a second opinion and found a fabulous neurologist who first wanted to take a look at my MRI. "Dont tell me anything yet. Let me take a look," she said.

She examined the scans for a few minutes and turned to me and said "Just looking at this and without knowing anything about your medical history, I'd say you have MS." From here we spoke in a lot more depth about the symptoms I'd experienced over the last few years and the sort of lifestyle I had.

It was her opinion I was living with a relapsing-remitting form of MS and we discussed a variety of treatment plans.

While having a definitive diagnosis was a load off my mind, reconciling the two different opinions of the neurologists I had seen was difficult. The first doctor said I didn't need to do anything and the second neurologist was recommending I start a drug treatment immediately. I was really emotional. I'm glad I had my sister with me at the appointment because I think I was in shock and I didn't really remember a lot about the treatment plan the neurologist was walking me through.

Despite some time lapsing between seeing those two different neurologists I didn't do a lot of research on MS. I found that doing a simple web search was more confusing than helpful. Unless you're a doctor the bulk of the information out there is very scientific and difficult to understand. Searching for information about 'benign MS' was just weird. It ended up confusing me more. The information was saying 'well you've got MS but at the moment it's just not active.' I was still having the dizzy spells so I couldn't understand how the disease wasn't active.

It helped me immensely to have found a supportive neurologist in the second opinion I sought; she was someone I could communicate with more easily and I also talked to MS Australia and they were really wonderful.

I'm not sure I'd say it was a relief to have a definitive diagnosis but it at least gave me something to work with. By this stage I had left my role in the bank and studied to become a fitness instructor. My husband and I had also moved from Melbourne and

I was now a full-time mum. Life was a little different to the first undiagnosed episode of MS five years earlier but the hamster wheel was still turning around furiously!

I would never sit down and take a few minutes to relax but after my diagnosis I realised I had to force myself to take time out at least once a day to just sit and rest. And particularly once the kids started school, I was on the go all day, so carving out a little bit of time to recharge my batteries became really important. Now, every day around lunch time, I make sure I sit down and eat properly and take a rest without feeling guilty. It took me a while to not look around and find other things to do, but now I know that if I don't take off that precious time between about 12 noon and 2pm I'll feel a lot worse later on in the day.

I guess when you're a mum you just think that you don't have time to be sick. I'd keep pushing through everything because I had the mindset that no one else was going to get everything done if I didn't.

This mindset was so challenging to overcome initially. I struggled with giving myself permission to take a break each day. Letting go of that feeling of having to get everything done feels a bit like losing control, but really it's all about gaining control; gaining control of your own time, health and wellbeing.

Early on my husband Paul couldn't read me as to how I felt or what sort of day I'd had. I guess I expected him to be able to read my mind because I certainly didn't want to have to confess to not feeling fabulous or to ask for help. Our mutual lack of understanding of the situation and what was required caused some tension between us and the first six months after my diagnosis were strained. I expected him to know what was going on without having to tell him and when he couldn't read the situation correctly or didn't know what to do, I became annoyed and angry.

I look back now and realise how much of an adjustment my diagnosis was for him. He hadn't known he was marrying a woman with MS and certainly had no prior experience caring for someone with a chronic illness. He was processing not only what it meant for him, but also our two daughters.

Eventually we worked out a little system for when he came home each night. I'd hold up a sign over my head that said 'good' or 'bad'! I realised that I had to either say something to Paul or give him the visual cues because he wasn't a mind reader and it wasn't fair to make him guess.

Frankly, my family was lost when having to deal with the diagnosis and it was a difficult transition for them. I think my father thought I was going to end up in a wheelchair for the rest of my life and I had to sit down with him and really explain what living with MS meant. In those early years he'd actually get fairly upset if I was having a bad day. I remember that on one of my off days I was lying down and I heard him explain to someone on the phone that they couldn't come over because I had MS that day! We joke about it now, but I had to spell out to him that I actually have MS every day... but some days it affects me worse than others.

Speaking with a psychologist helped me greatly in sorting through this early transition and I was able to better process what was going on. By being able to work through all these changes I could then communicate effectively with my husband and family. Giving the situation time and coming to an acceptance was also part of the process. I think both my husband and I came to the same conclusion at the same time as to what the situation was and that we just had to get on with life, albeit with some modifications.

I didn't want anyone to feel sorry for me and I didn't want to be known as 'Nic with MS.' I just wanted to be myself again. That sense of feeling out of control was really difficult. I like to be in control of everything but with the MS that's just not possible. My husband thinks it's pretty ironic that I now have to live with something that renders me unable to control everything!

I've learnt that having MS and being a mum means allowing yourself to ask for help. I have a great support group in my friends and family who I can turn to if I'm having an off day. Even simple things like having a friend pick up the girls from school so as I can take a longer rest or having my family do some jobs on the weekend is a great help. I don't have to try and do it all. It was hard but I've learnt I just need to accept the offer of help when I need it. It doesn't make me a lesser woman or mother. It allows me to build the strength to give back to my girls.

It was scary thinking about the future for my daughters; in fact it was one of the hardest things emotionally to consider and I guess you could say it was the driving force behind me maintaining a fit and healthy lifestyle so as I would be able to run around with them. There's so much I couldn't control about MS but I could control how I fuelled my body and how I kept it in good physical shape.

In the early days of living with my diagnosis I explored a lot of different dietary modifications. I tried cutting out gluten and dairy among other things, but for me, I came back to a really simple solution of eating a clean diet of unprocessed foods and a balanced combination of carbohydrates and proteins in every meal. I eat fruit and vegetables and drink lots of water and exercise every day, even if it's just a walk. Getting that little bit of rest every day is essential as well. If I follow this simple routine I just feel like I'm on top of the MS. If I deviate from this, as I sometimes do on the weekends, it can take my body three or four days to recover.

I've certainly looked at many of the other MS-advocated diets out there and while I'm not against them, I realised that my diet also needs to fit around looking after a young family. Making several variations of every meal proved to be more stressful for me than just finding a simple solution that suited - and nourished - the whole family. I've found my own solution and would encourage anyone living with MS to explore the variety of options and find the one that suits you and your lifestyle best. MS presents in a variety of ways and everyone's makeup and body is different, so to find a nutritional and exercise plan that suits your own situation is a better strategy to stressing out about whether you can stick to someone else's plan. Play around a little bit to figure out what your body responds favourably to and what you can also incorporate into your life, given your own unique working, living and energy situation.

While exercise, rest and nutrition have been the treatment that I control, I've also worked with my neurologist to explore a range of drug treatment options. Currently I'm on a drug trial that consists of an infusion I get when I do my annual MRI. This year we found that there have been no new lesions after taking the infusion over the last four years. This is good news but it's still really hard with MS to know what the body is doing. I often wonder whether my MS symptoms have been improved because of the drug treatment or whether it's because the MS is remitting. It can really play a mind trick with you. I think my day-to-day symptoms, such as the tingling feelings and some of the fatigue, seem to have decreased compared to when I wasn't on the trial but it can be hard to judge.

In coming to terms with the diagnosis I must admit I moped around a little. In fact there were some fairly shitty times. My husband and I are naturally fairly positive people but there was a lot to process and learn. Then there was this turning point where we both realised that the MS wasn't going anywhere and this was the life we were going to have to live so we might as well get on with things. We could both sit around feeling sorry for ourselves and let everything get on top of us or we could deal with whatever was going to come our way.

I don't know what finally made me decide to be positive but I just knew inherently it was the only way to be. I've met other people who went the other way and I decided it wasn't the way I wanted to deal with things. I didn't want to be defined by the illness. I want to make the most of life.

I don't want to mope around for my children to see either. I really believe that a positive attitude has played a huge role in how the MS affects me. I now surround myself with positive people. The few support groups I attended for chronically ill people were very depressing. I didn't want to be there talking about disability payments and health rebates. The meetings ended up making me feel guilty for wanting to be healthy and active and positive. Most of the people in the group were twenty years older than me and it was a bit confronting to think I might be that impaired eventually. I'm not trying to ignore what effects the MS may have on me as I age, but I'll deal with that when the time comes. I want to live in the 'now' and do what I can now to control the symptoms of the MS.

I believe in support groups but your support group could just as easily be made up of your girlfriends and family members. I get more from a coffee with my girlfriends on a bad day than the experience of the organised support group. I also find that because I have my own support group and they know about the MS I don't find the need to tell anyone else. When I go to events and functions where no one knows my history, I feel wonderfully free of the stigmas attached to having MS, and because I get to discuss it enough with my own support group, I don't have the need to bring it up with anyone else, so the MS doesn't end up defining me.

Another turning point for me was recognising that I had to let go of planning everything perfectly. Rarely do things ever go according to plan and allowing yourself to be flexible as to execution and outcomes is a key to successfully living with MS.

I had wanted to start my personal training business for years but when I was diagnosed with the MS I shelved the idea thinking I wouldn't be able to do it. I realised I was just using the condition as an excuse. It was dumb! I had no excuse. I had been using the MS as an excuse to not go ahead and plan anything for the future. It was when my daughters had finally started school and I was sitting at home with little to do that I realised I had nothing of me left. The girls had been my life and I'd been looking after them.

I was so passionate about health and fitness and helping others achieve it in their life and I really didn't have any excuses left to start the business. I also knew that I was probably not going to be the most reliable employee any longer, given my fatigue and those nasty 'off days,' so trying to shape a work environment that suited me was a good solution. To be honest, I don't know that I would ever have started my own business if it wasn't for the MS. I can look back now and say everything happens for a reason. It kind of sucks that it had

· 134 ·   TAKING CONTROL

to be MS, but I'm glad I had the courage to make the best of the situation.

It can be hard to make that initial decision on how to make those necessary life changes, but it comes down to doing what you need to do to prioritise your health. It's absolutely okay to look after yourself. I think we need to give ourselves permission to do this more often without feeling guilty about it. It's taken me some time to get my mind around it, but I know now that my health and well-being will be a priority forever.

Nicole's Top Tips

"The thing I found especially hard at the start was slowing down!"

Look after your body through exercise & nutrition: You don't know how many doctors, specialists, etc said to me "well you're fit and healthy. You're already better prepared than a lot of people." Take care of yourself by moving each day, whether it's through planned activity or incidental exercise - it all adds up. Also, think about everything you put into your mouth. OK, we're not always good ALL of the time but most of the time would be great start!

Knowledge is power: When I was first diagnosed in 2007 I didn't know anything about MS...except it was THAT disease where you ended up in a wheelchair! I read as much as I could to learn about my diagnosis. Learn through the internet, the MS society, books, support groups and doctors....the list goes on! I felt much better equipped knowing what I possibly might face in the future & what was happening to my body.

Plan: I always make sure I plan my whole day. And my day ALWAYS has a rest/sit down time during the middle of the day.

Support Group: The thing I found especially hard at the start was slowing down! And I never accepted anyone's help. Now I have an amazing group of friends and family that are always more than happy to help out in any way should I need them. Your own support group doesn't have to be a formal group you go to, it's just important to know who you can rely on and turn to for help or advice.

JEANIE MCMASTER

"When you have MS it's actually a bit isolating no matter where you live."

My diagnosis of MS literally crept up on me and completely took me by surprise. But I guess something like that could only ever be a surprise. I clearly remember feeling my first symptom. I woke up one morning and felt numb on both sides of my body from the waist down. It was a pretty scary thing to wake up to. I couldn't put the numbness down to anything in particular. I had been working hard in the gardens the day before but I knew I hadn't injured myself. The sensation frightened me enough to call my doctor immediately.

I live on a property about 20 minutes outside a small country town in north-west New South Wales called Warialda. We're lucky to have fabulous doctors out here, but attending to these types of symptoms would not be an everyday occurrence for them. Clem, one of the doctors, started suggesting all sorts of exotic conditions until he called his wife Di – who is the other GP - into the room. After reviewing my medical history and seeing that I'd had previous issues with my eyes, she raised the possibility of multiple sclerosis with me. I was referred to an ophthalmologist and then a neurologist on the Gold Coast.

I didn't mention it to Di and Clem at the time but looking back, I'd also been having some problems with my hands for a while.

Things would just fall through my fingers and I occasionally had difficulty picking up or grasping things.

So I found myself in a situation where I'm fine one day and then the next seeing specialists at a large city centre some six hours away. The neurologist scheduled me for an MRI. I'd never had one before and I hated it. I was trapped in a tube for an hour and a half and I just couldn't bear the noise. I didn't feel claustrophobic but instead overwhelmed by the clanging of the machine and the fact that I was left alone with nothing but dire thoughts. It was horrendous.

The MRI showed that I had lesions on my spine and brain and the neurologist performed a few more physical tests before confirming MS. At this point he felt that my MS was benign. The Johns Hopkins Multiple Sclerosis Center in Baltimore, America defines benign MS as a disease course where an individual will have mild disease after having MS for about 15 years. This occurs in about 5 to 10% of patients. There is no good way of predicting which patients will follow this course. The only way to identify benign MS is after someone has had the diagnosis of MS for at least 15 years and has had no evidence of worsening - both in functional ability and as evidenced on the MRI. Benign MS cannot be predicted at the time of diagnosis or even after a few years with MS.[5]

At this stage I was 48 and with the explanation my neurologist was giving me about benign MS I could look back and realise I'd been experiencing symptoms for quite some time. When I was 26 I had neuritis in my left eye and lost sight for probably a week and then about ten years later I also had a cataract in the same eye. Over the years I've had a lot of issues with that eye that I now thought to be various symptoms of this benign MS.

I felt a strange sense of relief at the information the neurologist had just given me. I knew that the condition could change over time but I no longer felt paranoid that I was going to be confined to a wheel chair immediately. I'm a bit like my mother in that respect. She was always a big advocate for finding out what was wrong and then just getting on with things. I also figured that I could only do what

I could do and that I just had to get on with my life.

It concerns me that the first thing we think of when we hear the phrase 'multiple sclerosis' is wheel chairs. I grew up in a time when one of our most notable Australian athletes was Betty Cuthbert, whom I hold a great deal of respect for. But most people would now associate her with being confined to a wheelchair because of her MS. I don't know why or how the image of a wheel chair is synonymous of MS but the way needs to be paved to associate living with MS with other inspirational things as it can be very frightening to picture yourself in a wheel chair the minute you're told you have MS.

Having spent the last few days in and out of hospitals and seeing specialists I just wanted to go home and get on with things. I wasn't too worried about how I would get treated or what resources where available because out here we're used to travelling to get what we need or simply living without it. I've always lived in a rural environment so what other people may see as isolation is actually fairly normal for me. I did end up changing to a neurologist who was only a two hour drive away rather than six but that's the only time I've made concessions to distance.

We have great GPs in town and I'm lucky to have such a close circle of friends who have become my support group. The only thing that does worry me on occasion is thinking what would happen if I had an accident or felt too sick to get help. I'm out on the property by myself a lot and I wonder who might eventually find me and how long that would take? But it's all relative. It could very well take me two hours and a lot of hassle to get to the doctor if I lived in the city between all the commuting, parking and navigating the large hospitals. And you could just as easily have an accident in a city apartment where no one finds you for weeks.

There are no formal support groups or MS clinics in Warialda but there are one or two other people I know who are also living with MS in the region and one of these women helped me quite a bit early on. We've had a few chats about diets and fatigue and things like that but what helped me the most was knowing that there was someone else close by who had MS. You just want to know there's someone else out there that can empathize with you. When you have MS it's actually a bit isolating no matter where you live. It's not a condition like cancer where a lot is known and everyone knows someone else with cancer. The lack of understanding and recognition around MS really annoys me. I can tell that no one really knows what to say to me (with regards to the MS) or how to help. People's interactions at times can be quite awkward.

I sometimes wonder what people think of me. When you're out in the sticks your business becomes everyone else's. My MS is not common knowledge but it's not a secret either. I'm sure people think I malinger every now and then or that I've been drinking if I'm a bit off balance. When I'm having a tough time with my MS symptoms I'll just stay at home for a few days and rest. I'll sort of hibernate rather than make excuses or explain what's going on. I find people don't actually realise that it's not always easy for me to just get stuck into things, which is what we're conditioned to do in the country.

I remember one of the locals coming up to me at a function I was attending and exclaiming how well I looked.

"It's great to see you've gotten over your MS Jeanie," he boomed. I don't get offended by those sorts of comments any longer. It actually amuses me. But he went on to say "And Jacqui looks well too!" Jacqui is a friend of mine also living with MS.

I find it amusing that we all seem to get put under the same banner but how do you educate people like that? I'm sure the comments are meant as a compliment but there is so little understanding around what MS actually is and I feel that people assume we're meant to look unwell. If I could wave my magic wand I'd wish for more understanding of MS. People need to realise that there are different forms and disease course. It affects people in different ways and we all live with it in different ways. One thing I can definitely say is that we don't all just end up in wheel chairs immediately, if at all. And we often look amazingly healthy even if we don't feel on top of the world.

I admit I find a lot of things to do with my MS really frustrating.

My loss of balance when I try to do simple things like put pants or socks on – that really annoys me. I might sit down to type on the computer and my hands don't want to work properly. Sometime you just feel really stunted in doing what you want to do. But you get on with it and get over it and in the end you find a way to make everything work.

I was never a terribly confident person; people might think I am but I'm not. Although over the years the MS has taken a little of my confidence away because I won't try to do things that I don't think I can do anymore. I just don't want to put myself in a position where I might hurt myself. Over the past five years or so I've found my strength and coordination has definitely changed. I used to be able to work in my client's gardens all day; lifting sleepers and rocks and digging holes. I certainly don't find it as easy any more. I really wonder how I did it back then.

I no longer ride horses either, which I'd love to do and I used to love surfing when I went to the coast, but I don't like to go into the waves anymore; that's just a waste of time getting knocked off your feet all the time!

And despite the fact that it sounds like I've had some of the things taken away from me that I used to love doing, I don't feel a void at all. I seem to have filled up those missing areas with other things that I now love to do. I entertain a lot more than I used to and I read a lot and do more things on the computer than I ever used to – for both work and entertainment.

It's a hard disease to have, because at times it can be very debilitating. My mind is not quite what it once was. My friends say they can't notice any difference but I know in myself that my mind isn't as sharp. Normal, everyday things just take that little bit more effort. From remembering birthdays through to the simple act of hopping in the car and driving, these all require a lot more thought and a lot more awareness and I get tired a lot more easily. But keep in mind, all these things I'm describing could be part of the act of aging; it just seems far more palatable to me to blame it on the MS instead.

I've become a lot more aware of how I manage my energy these days and I've become very protective of how I expend it. I can't cope with late nights so I tend to entertain over lunches instead. If I have friends staying I'll just crawl into bed when I need to but the thought of going to someone's place and staying until 3 o'clock in the morning fills me with horror because it's out of my control. Stress is probably the thing that saps my energy more than anything else though. That formula for managing your energy is an odd thing to try and pin down. It's finding that perfect balance to getting enough rest and living without stress, even though you can never live entirely without stress in life.

If you try to think of managing the MS in terms of everything being a trade off then I think you can actually get quite a bit accomplished. I'm very involved in the running of our local RNA Show and I can really put my heart and soul into it for a solid week but then I'll have to compensate by taking the week after the show off and recovering. It's the same with heat. I love summer weather and the sunshine but I can't stand the heat. There's a lot of internal negotiating to find the right outcome. One where you can still enjoy the things you love in life but also protect your health.

I figure the future will take care of itself. I don't want to end up in a wheelchair, but if that happens then so be it. I can't be worrying now about what the future may or may not bring with regards to my MS.

My thoughts around the future gravitate more towards aging gracefully. What I'd really like for the future is for a group of likeminded friends to buy a house, with lots of rooms, to hire a person who will look after us, cook us meals, pour us champagne in the afternoon and let us play cards all day. There would always be someone to have a laugh with, to go to the movies with, just so long as there's someone there to cook and clean and the nurses to give us our pills on time!

Jeanie's Tips for Making Life Easier with MS

- I tend to eat a fairly clean and light diet, generally free of saturated fats. So one thing I've learnt to do when I crave a little bit of red meat, such as a roast dinner is to invite friends around for dinner. That way there's no leftovers and I can really enjoy it.

- I really enjoy the companionship, responsibility and exercise you get from owning a pet.

CORINDA MCNAUGHTON

"I've had nearly five years of living with MS now and to be honest, it has made me realise that I can do anything."

In the time leading up to my initial episode of MS, I didn't think my life was any more or less stressful than anyone else's. Two years earlier I had given birth to two beautiful twin girls and between raising them and working part time I was constantly on the go. About six weeks before my diagnosis I'd also suffered chicken pox and then gastro, so perhaps my body was trying to tell me something after all!

I had been experiencing blinding headaches for about three weeks and even though I'd been back to the doctor several times we hadn't been able to get rid of them. The doctor believed I just had a really bad migraine and needed to let it run its course. But it just didn't feel like that at all. I was tired and stressed and still working three days a week at that point. Between work and the kids everything was just getting on top of me. But after weeks of enduring these headaches I couldn't stand the pain any longer and went back to the doctor.

He still didn't believe it was anything more serious than a migraine and suggested I get a massage. I explained to him that I felt like my eye balls were going to explode out of my head; that's how tremendous the pressure was behind my eyes. Still, he maintained I merely had a bad migraine and told me to go home and return in another week if it got any worse. At this point I felt like I was being fobbed off.

So a few days later I was with the kids at playgroup and just felt really strange. I had started losing sight in one eye and I decided to go and see an optometrist immediately.

He had me take a few different vision tests and to the alarm of both the optometrist and myself I couldn't read anything. He immediately referred me to another eye specialist in Melbourne.

This specialist discovered that my optic nerve was incredibly swollen and he wanted me to additionally consult a neurologist to see what was causing the swelling. At this point I started to become quite concerned. Whatever was going on was no longer an inconvenience - it was starting to get scary. The ophthalmologist said a best case scenario would be that I had MS or at worst case I had a tumour on my optical nerve or a brain tumour. What a trio to choose from!

Within days I was consulting with a neurologist in Melbourne for an MRI and lumbar puncture. I knew deep down after I had the MRI that I had multiple sclerosis but I still had to wait four weeks for the results of the lumbar puncture to come back in. They finally told me a week before my 32nd birthday that I had MS and it took me four weeks to regain my sight and a further three months to recover from this initial episode.

Before all this exploration I didn't know anything about MS. All I was thinking was that I was doomed and that I was going to end up in a wheelchair. I started going through a massive amount of grief. I urged my husband to take the kids and find a better life for themselves. I went through a very rough patch where I just didn't really want to live and thought I was being punished for something. I truly believed the world hated me.

I remember one day, early after the diagnosis, that I just lay on the kitchen floor screaming and crying. My husband came and sat with me and tried to calm me down.

"What's wrong Corinda?" he asked.

"I can't do this," I said. "You can't see it, but I feel like I'm dying from the inside out. I just don't know what to do; I don't know how to fix this." I felt like I had the pieces of the jigsaw but couldn't make them fit together to complete the picture. Life just looked like a big unsolvable puzzle at that point.

I felt this horrible guilt and despair for at least 12 months. It felt like I was just existing – not actually living life at all. I guess the reality of the situation hit me harder than I thought. One of my biggest anxieties in life was change. I'd always had a huge fear of it and at the time of my diagnosis I was constantly saying 'what if?' Like 'what if I can't work anymore?' or 'what if we don't have enough money?'

But maybe because I'd finally broken down in tears and let some of the anger go, something clicked. I realised that life is too short. My husband said he'd rather do something and regret doing it than not have done something at all.

The first medication my neurologist had me on felt so bad that I decided I'd rather come off it and have five good years with my kids than stay on it and suffer every day. I put up with it for two years but one thing led to another and I actually didn't take any meds for about six months. I went through a phase were I actually felt really good. I figured that if I felt that good then clearly I didn't have MS any more. Maybe I was just pretending that the MS didn't really exist. I finally confessed to my neurologist that I hadn't been taking my medication but I was clearly okay for not taking anything. He just rolled his eyes and said we should let an updated MRI scan be the real judge.

So I had that MRI and that's when my world fell apart again. I had four new lesions on my brain, one in my spinal cord and one in my neck.

I felt so stupid. In hindsight I couldn't understand why I thought being off my medication would be a good thing. While my neurologist didn't get mad at me the situation at least opened the discussion for working out an alternative treatment plan because the current medication was making me miserable. After a lot of research and consideration I eventually changed to another medication and have been successfully taking that for over two years now.

MS treatments don't cure MS, but they can be effective at helping reduce the frequency of relapses. Some treatments have been proven to help slow the progression of MS, while others are designed to alleviate certain symptoms.

When considering your treatment options it's important to work with your healthcare team early to define your goals. Once you have a clear idea of what you can realistically expect from your therapy, you and your healthcare team can create the treatment plan that's right for you.

When evaluating MS treatment options, there are a number of choices. They all have different benefits, side effects, dosing schedules and routes of administration. MS clinics around the world have access to specially trained MS nurses that can assist you in finding the right information in conjunction with your neurologist.

"MS does not define the person I am."

Since my diagnosis I've had to learn to let go of things. I'm a much more positive person now. In the past I was always worried about everything and was the world's best at making excuses for not giving things a go. I was always trying to solve other people's problems and at the same time worrying if I should have done things differently. I was probably the most pessimistic person you could meet. If I could blame someone else for a problem, I would. A friend could say "It's a beautiful day today." And I'd reply "Yeah, but it's too hot." I'd turn anything into a negative.

Maybe being diagnosed with MS was the 'Big Guy Upstairs' way of making me realise that I had to start being nice to myself. Now I realise that thinking pessimistically is just not good for me. As strange as it sounds, getting MS has taught me that I can stand on my own two feet and make decisions I live with. Maybe it's because I understand that I need to look after myself and my interests now and that realisation is sort of empowering. In a lot of ways I feel like my diagnosis has allowed me to make a clean start.

Before my diagnosis I hated change yet since then I have moved to the other side of the country and away from my family and close friends. I started living the life I want to live and I've never been happier.

My psychologist was my saviour. She pushed me to mental and emotional boundaries that forced me to examine my negative beliefs. I clearly remember that light bulb moment when I cried into my hands one day saying to her "Why me? What did I do to be given MS?"

I had in my brain that getting MS was a punishment for something I had done wrong. She simply replied "why not you?" That realisation that it could happen to anyone and the 'it' could actually be far, far worse, gave me a new perspective. Now I don't consider MS to be the death sentence I once thought it was. It's the wake up call to go and live my life whether people approve of the way I live it or not. I owe it to myself, my husband and my children to be the best I can be, MS or not. MS does not define the person I am.

"I was out to prove to people that I could still do it."

I had been working as a florist three days a week prior to my diagnosis and I also had very young children. Eventually I decided to resign as I just couldn't do the floristry work standing on my feet for eight to ten hours a day any longer. I was exhausted and my children were suffering because of it.

Around this time I decided to apply for the MS Australia 'Go for Gold Scholarship.' I was initially a bit reluctant to apply because I hadn't spent a lot of time around other people with MS and if I was lucky enough to receive it I would be thrust into that environment. Maybe it was just my own coping technique, but I didn't really want to talk about MS or learn about it, otherwise my own situation might become a bit too real. But the funny thing is I was awarded the scholarship in 2008 and I eventually started reading some of the Society's magazines and ended up at a few MS Society functions where I met wonderful people and learned many really great ways of treating and coping with MS.

So with my newly minted mindset of cleaning the slate I figured I could reinvent myself a bit more through the scholarship and learn new skills. And because I now had a disability I could see how disadvantaged others with disabilities were. I'd always wanted to help out kids in a classroom and I thought if I had a kid with a disability I'd want all the help I could get. So with my scholarship I chose to go back to university and study to become an integration aid.

Going back to university was so empowering. I hadn't studied for many years but it was really good for me to figure out different ways to do things and to think outside the box. I was out to prove to people that I could still do it. I wanted people to know that regardless of the fact I had MS I could absolutely still go out and achieve things.

> ### *"There's always a solution to every problem."*

It's a doubled edged sword sometimes, having MS. Of course I want to remain independent and active in life but there are times when I need the assistance or decline to do things because of the heat or lack of energy. It can be difficult for the people around us to judge how to handle that situation and it can be equally difficult for us not to become frustrated if we just can't do what we want to do and at the time we've chosen.

The other thing is that because MS affects everyone differently, we all look different. There's no one defining characteristic that screams 'You've got MS.' The standard image of a person with MS is one in a wheelchair. I hate being lumped into that category. We need more awareness and education of the general public as to what MS is and the range of ways it can affect people and how best to offer support.

I've learnt that managing my MS is a daily trade-off. You have a certain amount of energy to give out and you have to use it wisely. I still do the things I love to do, but I have to choose wisely when and how I'm going to do them or know that I'm going to pay for it in an energy deficit the next day. But there's always a solution to every problem.

Learning to say no to people has been one of the hardest skills to learn. But you have to work out the activities that work for you and those that will have a negative effect. In the early days I used to really worry about saying 'no' to people; it would bother me for days. One day my psychologist asked me why I put so much effort into worrying about what other people thought.

"Do you think they go home after you've said no to something and lie awake analysing your decision all night?" she enquired. That sentiment put it all into perspective for me!

I've had nearly five years of living with MS now and to be honest, it has made me realise that I can do anything. It's made me much more determined than ever and I am emotionally stronger than I have been in years. I have a new-found confidence and try not to let things get me down any longer.

Corinda's Tips for Living with MS:

"I owe it to myself, my husband and my children to be the best I can be - MS or not. In no way does MS define the person I am."

Social Networking Sites: I've personally found Facebook really helpful in making connections with other people living with MS. There are plenty of Facebook groups and pages out there with the common thread of MS and you're bound to be able to find a group that has other like minded people. Over the last few years I've corresponded with people from all around the world and made some really good friends. It can certainly be less confronting than a formal support group.

Inspirational Reads: Whenever I feel a bit down I have a collection of 'go to' books I like to read. They never fail to bring a new perspective or cheer me up. My current picks are Paul Coelho's 'The Alchemist,' Elizabeth Gilbert's 'Eat Pray Love,' and I've also just started reading Nick Vujicic's 'Life Without Limits.' I love being able to get a positive lesson from a good story!

Get Informed: Read and research and educate yourself as much as you can. Only then can you make informed decisions. You will be hit with so much information on health and well being – let alone MS – and from a variety of people, so it's important that you have a s much knowledge as possible so you can navigate your way through all the information and decide what is best for you.

HAZEL MOREL

"I can't change what has happened to me but even though I have a disability, I feel like I'm living a life much like anyone else's now."

....

Currently more than 7,500 young Australians with full-time care needs are living in aged care facilities simply because there are few alternatives. There are also 700,000 more young Australians being cared for at home by family and friends, often with limited support. [6]

Many have long lives to live, yet the realities of aged care mean they will share a residence where the average age is 83.5 and the average length of stay less than three years.

Being young is about having a lifetime ahead of you, yet aged care is designed for someone who is at the end of their life. In most cases, the specific care needs of a young person will not be met in aged care as they differ greatly to those of the elderly residents.

The statistics for those young people living in aged care are startling:

- 44% will receive a visit from friends less than once a year
- 34% will almost never participate in community based activities such as shopping
- 21% will go outside the home less than once a month. [7]

Responding to this dire situation was one inspirational young woman. Youngcare was formed in 2005 when Shevaune Conry, herself living with MS, found that her care needs became too great for her to remain at home in the care of her loved ones. Despite the best efforts of her family and friends to care for her, they discovered her only option was to live in aged care.

Shevaune uncovered a desperate lack of full-time care options for young people in Australia. To her it was truly shocking and devastating. This enormous injustice sparked Shevaune's loved ones - David Conry, Matt Lawson, Simon Lockyer and Nick Bonifant to co-found Youngcare, vowing to change the way young people are cared for.

Shevaune's story literally moved thousands of supportive Australians including businesses, government and the community, resulting in the construction of the first ever Youngcare Apartments in 2007. Shevaune moved out of aged care and into her very own apartment, along with 15 other young people with high care needs. Finally, change had occurred – an example of what could be done – and Shevaune had a home that provided all the care and support she needed, enabling her to live the young life she so rightly deserved.

Sadly Shevaune passed away in 2012 but her work is recognised as being pivotal in creating modern-day change in Australia's social fabric; for creating big, bright sparks of hope in the homes of many families right across the nation and proved that change is absolutely possible in this lifetime for young people in desperate need of real care accommodation options.

For many residents of the Youngcare Apartments around Australia, their life is now a lot brighter because of access to supported housing options. One such person is Hazel and this is her story.

***

I was diagnosed with MS when I was 21, which is twenty years ago now. I clearly remember my first symptoms coming on suddenly and from nowhere. I couldn't see out of my right eye at all and I also had some numbness down one side of my body. Although I have to admit I thought the numbness was because I'd fallen asleep at night with my electric blanket on even though mum had warned me not to! Dad called the doctor - thinking I might have been getting glaucoma – and she quickly referred my to an eye specialist who then referred me to a neurologist. After a few days in hospital, where they did EEG tests and a lumbar puncture, it was confirmed that I had relapsing-remitting MS.

It was a lot of information for a twenty year old to comprehend but I must have just taken it into my stride. I don't think I really knew what else to do other than to just get on with things.

And that's just what I did. For the first decade I lived life to the fullest. I had a successful career in the travel industry; I got married and also had a son. Those first ten years were full of changes but in your 20s and 30s that's what life is about.

I had some time off after having my son and I actually felt really great. The specialists put it down to the fact that my hormones were very active and carrying me along. To be honest I felt like I could do just about anything and I eventually went back to work after 12 months of maternity leave. But this was short-lived. Maybe I was too ambitious thinking I could manage a full-time workload and also raise a child or maybe it was just the effects of ten years of MS on the body, but I only lasted three months before I needed to resign. I was just exhausted and I felt like I was becoming physically and cognitively slower at everything.

At this point I also felt that I should take myself off the road. Because of the loss of sensation in my legs my reactions whilst driving weren't up to par and I felt that for the safety of my son and others on the road I needed to stop driving. Around the same time my sense of balance also became very poor. I could just feel a real change in my body. My relapsing-remitting MS had displayed fairly regular patterns over the years of flaring up for two months at a time and then settling right down for many months. Now however, some of the symptoms weren't going away and the flares were happening more regularly.

I consulted my neurologist about this decline and an MRI confirmed that the lesions in my brain had also spread into my spine.

At the time my neurologist was Professor Pender, a world-renowned researcher of MS. After examining all my symptoms and the scans, he felt that my disease course had moved into secondary progressive MS. I was actually really thankful when Professor Pender broke this news to me. I just wanted someone to admit what I already knew: That my body had changed for good. Up until then everyone had been beating around the bush and treating me with kid gloves when really all I wanted was the truth. If I had the truth I knew what I was dealing with.

Not long after this I also switched to using a wheelchair full time. I just found it easier to get around as I didn't have the energy to go great distances in the walker any more. However I still had fairly good use of my hands at this point and an occupational therapist encouraged me to adapt to driving in a car with hand controls. It took me about five lessons to learn how to do it but I was then able to convert my licence over and this enabled me to retain a fair bit of independence. I could still drive my son to school and being able to drive was actually quite a relief when everything else around me was changing.

Unfortunately my marriage broke down in 2007. One of the Youngcare counsellors told me that 70% of all relationships involving the care of a young person with full-time care needs will end in divorce and this in fact is where the greatest impact is felt. In many cases it is not just the individual requiring care that is in crisis. Certainly my breakup brought a great deal of changes. One of these was that I no longer had a car and I felt like all my independence had been taken away. Losing that little bit of independence was so heart breaking and I found it very difficult to have to learn to rely on other people to get around. Not having a car may sound like a small and insignificant thing but it made a huge impact on my life.

By the next year my funding for at-home care had also run out and I realised that now I had to make some hard decisions on how I was going to live and be cared for. At that stage my son was still living primarily with me but spending weekends with his dad.

One of my biggest goals in life is to be the best mother that I can, but I found a complete lack of options available for a young mum with a disability to be able to continue living in a meaningful and dignified way.

Luckily I was sent a lifeline and was offered one of the first Young-care Apartments after they were finished construction. Living here has allowed me to continue being a mum. In comparison to an aged care facility, my apartment is a much more practical and cheerful place to have my son stay and he even has his friends over to visit when he's here – just like he would if we were still living at home. He can stay here with me on the weekends and in school holidays and we can do things as a family now, such as going to a concert, seeing a movie or catching a footy game.

When I first moved in five years ago I was a complete stranger and never thought I'd get to know everyone or get used to the new environment. Now it really is my home and my friendships with the other residents mean the world to me. The funny thing is the strong relationships you build with people you've never met before and would never think you could become friendly with but there's a special bond between everyone. They're like family now.

I feel mentally and physically stronger living here. We have activities every day that keep us active and it might sound a bit like summer camp, but these things are really important so as you don't feel like parts of your life are being taken away. Every day there's something to keep my brain active and I'm not sure that would have been the case in an aged-care facility. Over the last few years I've gotten very interested in skincare and cosmetics and I've been able to set up my own business here as a Nutrimetric's rep. It's so rewarding to be able to be able to extend my horizons and continue to make some income for myself.

My love of travel and adventure is still indulged too. I'm able to take my son away on vacation and there's always someone at the centre willing to take a cruise or overseas trip. I think because

I always have people around me now I don't feel isolated and still have the confidence to get out into the world.

The support network and on-site medical help has eliminated a great deal of stress in life and as anyone with MS knows, we need to try and reduce as much stress as possible. And always having someone to talk to is tremendously important to keeping mentally and emotionally strong.

I can't change what has happened to me but even though I have a disability, I feel like I'm living a life much like anyone else's now.

***

Youngcare works to deliver greater choice through four main programs:

Youngcare housing: To provide dignified and age-appropriate options in supported accommodation. Currently, there are two Youngcare Apartment buildings located in Brisbane and at the Gold Coast, with a third project underway in Sydney.

Youngcare Connect: A national information and support hotline. This service assists to connect young people and their families to relevant information and programs within government and the broader health care system.

Youngcare At Home Care Grants: For the provision of essential support items such as hoists, speech recognition devices, respite care and renovations to make homes disability friendly; to ultimately help young people with fulltime care needs stay at home for as long as possible in the care of loved ones and prevent a future in aged care.

Youngcare Research: In partnership with Griffith University – We are working more comprehensively to understand the needs and wants of young people with high care needs.

www.youngcare.com.au

Hazel's Tips:

- Don't ever give up. It's not the be all and end all.
- You may have a disability now but it shouldn't make you different to others.
- Keep doing everything that you can do while you can keep doing them – never let an opportunity pass.
- Take the diagnosis into your stride and try to never over-extend yourself. It just takes longer to recover if you do.

EMPLOYMENT, SUPERANNUATION AND INSURANCE

Guidance for people with Multiple Sclerosis

....

Adiagnosis of MS can change a person's life in many ways. For most people, even though they may have been diagnosed with MS, they are still able to work for many years post their original diagnosis. For others, their work capacity can be affected in the short term, sometimes immediately.

It is essential that anyone diagnosed with MS understands their legal rights regarding employment and superannuation so that they can maximise their chance of remaining in the work force and organise their financial affairs so that if they have to stop work because of their MS, they are not in a serious financial predicament.

Sometimes a minor change, such as a reduction in working hours can have a devastating impact on someone's superannuation and insurance entitlements.

Before making any decisions, anyone diagnosed with MS should ensure that they speak to an expert about their employment and superannuation.

Employment issues, Discrimination, Disclosure and MS:

Generally, you don't have to tell your employer about your condition unless it's relevant to the job or an occupational health and safety risk. It's important to assess what the reaction of your employer will be and to seek advice on this. In many cases telling your employer is a positive move - it may help explain any problems you are having at work and may result in changes to help you continue to work productively.

If you don't get a job or insurance cover because of your disability, you may have adiscrimination claim. Employers must take reasonable steps to accommodate their employees' disabilities, including changing your work environment, allowing time off for medical treatment, changing work duties in some circumstances and allowing you to work part-time. If your employer won't help, you may have a legal claim under anti-discrimination or workplace laws.

If you think you will be stopping work, you might be eligible for employment termination payments. The amount you get paid may depend on why you leave work and whether it's voluntary or not.

If you believe that you have been unfairly treated in the workplace, you should contact the MS Society, your union, or Maurice Blackburn Lawyers' Disability Helpline for advice.

Superannuation, Insurance and Employment entitlements:

Almost all employment superannuation funds offer disability insurance that covers you if you are no longer able to work due to MS. Many people also have private insurance, and sometimes an employer takes out insurance cover for all or some of their employees.

The common types of insurance are Total and Permanent Disability (TPD) insurance, income protection (I.P.) insurance, Trauma insurance and Life insurance (sometimes called death insurance).

TPD Insurance:

TPD insurance can vary greatly, but ordinarily covers you if you are no longer able to do your job, or any other job that you are reasonably trained or qualified for. You do not have to be unable to do all work, just work using your knowledge and transferrable skills. For example, if you've only ever done manual work, it won't matter if the doctors say you could do office work.

The amount of your insurance cover usually changes depending on your age and reduces as you get older, but not always. The insurance benefits are usually paid as a once off lump sum. The insurance benefits are often worth hundreds of thousands of dollars, and sometimes, although rarely, more than a million dollars.

If you have super funds from old jobs you might have continuing insurance cover even though you are on longer paying money into that fund. You can have more than one TPD claim so it is important to check what super funds you have and get advice before consolidating your super.

Income Protection Insurance:

Income Protection insurance is usually paid as a monthly benefit to replace your income. The amount of your entitlement varies greatly depending on your insurance policy. Often an income protection insurance policy will pay you up to 75% of your pre-disability earnings if you are unable to work.

Income Protection benefits are usually paid for 2 years. Some policies will pay benefits until age 65, or even the rest of your life.

Some superannuation funds offer income protection insurance that will cover you if your MS means that you can't work for the time being. Even if you had MS at the time that you joined the super fund, you will usually still be able to claim.

Income Protection insurance policies can vary greatly from policy to policy and it is important to get advice before making any decisions regarding your work hours. A reduction in your work hours may affect your entitlements.

Trauma Insurance:

Trauma insurance is an increasingly common type of insurance. Some Trauma insurance will usually pay you simply because you have been diagnosed with MS. Some policies will require that you have a particular level of impairment before you would be entitled to be paid, for example, 25% whole person impairment.

Again, trauma policies can vary greatly and it is important to get expert advice before lodging a claim.

How can I get Insurance cover if I have MS?

It is usually hard for people to get personal disability insurance cover if they have been diagnosed with MS. However, it may be possible to get insurance cover through an employment super fund.

Many employment super funds offer insurance cover to you as a member without the need for any health disclosure. This means that when you join an employment super fund, you are usually automatically covered for a base level of Death and TPD insurance that will cover you even if you have to stop work due to MS.

All super funds, have different insurance arrangements (or sometimes no insurance at all), and have different rules. It is really important that you get advice to ensure that you understand your entitlements before making any decisions. These issues can sometimes be complex and it is worth speaking to an expert.

What if an insurer or super fund rejects my claim?

If a super fund or insurer rejects your claim, you have rights of appeal.

If a claim is rejected, then you can lodge a complaint and request that the insurer or super fund review their original decision. If the insurer or super fund rejects your complaint or if you're mucked around, then you can apply to the Financial Ombudsman Service or the Superannuation Complaints Tribunal, or you can lodge a claim with a Court.

If your claim is rejected or if you are mucked around it is very important to get expert advice. These matters are not straight forward and it is worth getting someone who knows what they are doing to have a look at it.

Checklist

If any of the following apply, please get advice about your employment, superannuation and insurance rights BEFORE you do anything.

- If you have already stopped work because of MS;
- If you are thinking of stopping work because of MS;
- If you want to change your work hours or duties because of MS;
- If you are worried your employer might sack you;
- If you have been offered or might be offered a redundancy;
- If you are thinking of changing jobs or returning to work;

Free Advice:

This information was kindly provided by Paul Watson, a lawyer in the Superannuation & Insurance Claims group at Maurice Blackburn who is passionate about the rights of disabled and injured people. Paul, along with John Berrill, the head of the national Superannuation & Insurance Claims department, has developed many resources for the disability sector to assist them in understanding their rights.

Paul often runs seminars for disability support groups, social workers and medical professionals and is familiar with the issues faced by people with a disability.

Maurice Blackburn Lawyers has set up a free Australian service called the Disability Helpline (1800 196 050). The Disability Helpline is a free service to ensure that people can find out what their rights and entitlements are, without charge.

REFERENCES

1. Page 77: National MS Society. http://tinyurl.com/ks8rbk
2. Page 78: National MS Society. http://tinyurl.com/cvpy26z
3. Page 91: National MS Society. http://tinyurl.com/3patotf
4. Page 127: National MS Society. http://tinyurl.com/boefuo9
5. Page 138: Johns Hopkins Medicine. http://tinyurl.com/c3532t9
6. Page 155: Australian Institute of Health & Welfare 2007
7. Page 155: Di Winkler et al Winkler, D., L. Farnworth, et al. (2006). Australian Health Review.

ACKNOWLEDGEMENTS

Writing acknowledgements is a bit like delivering an Oscar's speech I imagine and there's always the risk I'll forget someone. However I can say first and foremost that my family have been my 'everything.' My Mum and my Dad have suffered unbelievable pain throughout my diagnosis of both MS and then breast cancer and they held it together for me. They have supported and encouraged me to develop this book series and help me believe in myself even when I wasn't so sure. My sister Rachel, also a journalist, offered endless support and suggestions and never once let me down. Her ideas have made this a stronger concept.

A huge thanks to each and every person I interviewed for this book; for laying your souls bare and trusting me with your story. Regan, Hayley, Alex, Nicole, Dianne, Linda, Tim, Paul, Corinda, Jeanie and Hazel you will be friends for life and I thank you for the strength and inspiration you have all given me.

To Kaye Hooper and Paul Watson who have provided such wonderful material in their forewords and legal resources chapter respectively. You are both wonderfully empathetic people who work tirelessly for patients and families dealing with MS.

And to Gerard Benjamin, a fellow writer, for offering philosophical guidance, technical expertise and sage encouragement over our monthly cups of coffee.

***

If you enjoyed this book you may be interested
in the next two books in the series.

Book 2 will talk to the carers of people with MS - be it their
mother, father, husband, wife, children or professional carer.

Book 3 will currate the knowldge of MS Nurses from
around the world. Their unique insight into dealing and living
with MS will provide valuable information to
patients and families alike.

www.take20stories.com

www.ingramcontent.com/pod-product-compliance
Lightning Source LLC
Chambersburg PA
CBHW020545270326
41927CB00006B/728